Implementing the National Service Framework for Coronary Heart Disease in Primary

Radcliffe Medical Press

£19.95

Radcliffe Medical Press
18 Marcham Road, Abingdon, Oxon OX14 1AA

British Library Cataloguing in Publication Data

A catalogue record for this book is available from the British Library.

ISBN 1 85775 506 5

Typeset by Joshua Associates Ltd, Oxford
Printed and bound by TJ International Ltd, Padstow, Cornwall

Contents

Foreword

The National Service Frameworks (NSFs) offer the promise of high-quality standardised care irrespective of where you live or who is responsible for local health and services. It has been said that of all the NSFs, the NSF for Coronary Heart Disease will be the most visibly easy to deliver – partly because it covers a specific disease area and partly because its aspirations are both equally specific and measurable.

But an NSF can achieve little on its own. It depends upon the skills, motivation and resources of those whose job it is to deliver it, particularly those working in primary care, who can have the most impact upon death and illness due to coronary heart disease. Hence this book, which will be a valuable companion for all those who are leading the revolution in coronary heart disease prevention and treatment in primary care today.

The text is packed with information that summarises current evidence in an easily usable form. Where possible, the theory is backed up by living examples of what is already being achieved in the field. It is, above all, a practical book, written very much from the perspective of primary care professionals, primary care teams and primary care organisations, with plenty of useful advice and suggestions as to how each might play a useful role in implementing the NSF. It is, however, more than simply a compendium of information, advice and useful tips. It stresses, quite rightly, that delivery of the NSF must be set in the context of effective systems for clinical governance and a culture which encourages continuous professional development.

One of the most interesting developments in the New NHS has been the convergence of primary care, secondary care and public health. The meeting of all three is long overdue, and it promises a new collective approach to commissioning and provision spiced with creative tension. It is particularly apt therefore that the authors of this book originate from each of these disciplines – but it is more than a symbolic partnership. Together they have created a piece of work that will both inspire and enable primary care to deliver the NSF for Coronary Heart Disease.

Michael Dixon
Chair, NHS Alliance
May 2001

About the authors

Zafar Iqbal entered public health medicine after completing a general practice vocational training scheme in 1989. He became a public health consultant at South Staffordshire Health Authority in 1994, and is currently also an honorary senior lecturer in public health medicine at Birmingham University. In the last few years Zafar has recommenced his career in general practice on a sessional basis.

He is currently leading the implementation of the coronary heart disease National Service Framework within South Staffordshire, and is a member of the West Midlands Regional Cardiac Forum. In recent years he has been involved in a variety of initiatives to promote a more systematic approach to the management of this chronic disease in the primary care setting. Zafar's other main interest is clinical governance and the way in which this links in with delivering the National Service Frameworks.

Ruth Chambers has been a GP for 20 years and is currently the professor of primary care development at Staffordshire University. She is the national education lead for the NHS Alliance. Ruth has designed and organised many types of educational initiatives, including distance-learning programmes. Recently she has developed a keen interest in working with GPs, nurses and others in primary care around clinical governance and practice personal and professional development plans. She is co-authoring a new series of books designed to help readers draw up their own personal development plan or practice learning plan around important clinical topics, such as coronary heart disease.

Paul Woodmansey qualified in medicine from Sheffield University in 1986, having received an intercalated B Med Sci degree. He became a member of the Royal College of Physicians in 1989, and was made a Fellow in 2000. His publications have included papers on coronary thrombolysis and pulmonary hypertension, the latter leading to the award of an MD in 1995. In the same year he was appointed as a consultant cardiologist to the Mid Staffordshire NHS Hospitals Trust. He is the clinical lead for implementation of the National Service Framework for coronary heart disease for the trust. He liaises between secondary and primary care and has written guidelines for both sectors.

Acknowledgements

We should like to thank the following people for a variety of contributions, including ideas, data and reference material:

- Paula Williams, Library Services Manager and Researcher, South Staffordshire Health Authority
- Andrew Lavelle, Information Analyst, South Staffordshire Health Authority
- Dr Mike Wall, Director of Public Health, South Staffordshire
- Chris Oliver, Clinical Development Facilitator for the CHD NSF at Queens Hospital Burton and East Staffordshire Primary Care Group
- Rosie Jones, Health Care Development Manager, Burntwood/ Lichfield Primary Care Group
- Christine Fearns, CHD NSF Co-ordinator, Birmingham Health Authority
- Dr Adrian Parkes, Clinical Governance Lead, Tamworth Primary Care Group
- Dr Tom Marshall, Lecturer, Department of Public Health and Epidemiology, University of Birmingham
- Jane Powell, Regional CHD Co-ordinator, NHS West Midlands Partnership for Developing Quality
- Dr Gill Wakley, GP, and co-author with Ruth Chambers of several books on clinical governance and continuing professional development.

We could not have completed the book without the continuing support and encouragement at home from Hifsa Iqbal and Chris Chambers, and the help of our amazing secretaries, Pam and Barbara.

List of abbreviations

ACE	angiotensin-converting enzyme
AF	atrial fibrillation
BMI	body mass index
BP	blood pressure
CABG	coronary artery bypass grafting
CHD	coronary heart disease
CPD	continuing professional development
CVA	cerebrovascular accident
CVD	cardiovascular disease
FPG	fasting plasma glucose
ECG	electrocardiogram
HA	health authority
HAZ	Health Action Zone
HDL	high-density lipoprotein
HF	heart failure
Hg	mercury
HImP	health improvement programme
IHD	ischaemic heart disease
INR	international normalised ratio
IT	information technology
LA	local authority
LDL	low-density lipoprotein
MAAG	medical audit advisory group
MI	myocardial infarction
NHS	National Health Service
NNS	number needed to screen
NNT	number needed to treat
NRT	nicotine replacement therapy
NSF	National Service Framework
NYHA	New York Heart Association
PCG	primary care group
PCO	primary care organisation
PCT	primary care trust
PTCA	percutaneous transluminal coronary angioplasty
PVD	peripheral vascular disease
RCT	randomised controlled trial
SIGN	Scottish Intercollegiate Guidelines Network
TIA	transient ischaemic attack
WHO	World Health Organisation

Introduction – focus continuing professional development on coronary heart disease

Coronary heart disease (CHD) is the single commonest cause of death in the UK, and much of the ensuing morbidity and premature mortality is preventable. Reducing the death rate from coronary heart disease, stroke and related diseases in people under 75 years old by at least 40% would save up to 200 000 lives – the target set by the English government for 2010.[1] The National Service Framework (NSF) for coronary heart disease[2] for England sets out milestones and goals for the health service.

We are using the term 'primary care organisation' (PCO) in this book to include every primary care group/trust in England. However, the material in the book is relevant to the provision of high-quality coronary heart disease care and services in local health groups in Wales, local health care co-operatives in Scotland and local health and social care groups in Northern Ireland, but the National Service Framework requirements for CHD only apply to England.

This book is written for primary healthcare teams and those working in primary care organisations, to help GPs, nurses and practice managers to implement the National Service Framework for coronary heart disease. It is also an essential resource for public health physicians and nurses and clinical governance leads who are responsible for implementing the NSF for CHD in their local area.

You can work through the book as an individual, as a practice team or as a few practices working together. There are many practical tips for improving the quality of coronary heart disease care and services in practice.

Practice teams need to develop a dual focus on improving the clinical management of coronary heart disease and improving the efficiency of their working environment. Team members should work together to direct their individual personal learning plans to form their practice personal and professional development plan. This should complement the clinical governance and business plans of the practice or primary care organisation.[3]

The NSFs for England give a clinical focus to strategic development of the health service. NSFs aim to improve standards and the quality of care, and to reduce variations in services. The national standards set out in the NSF for coronary heart disease will be delivered through clinical governance and local health improvement programmes. The NSFs have a strong patient focus, including provision of good information, opportunities for patients to participate in decision making, and more transparency about service quality and outcomes. Delivery is underpinned by professional self-regulation, research and development into effective interventions, and support for an increasingly skilled work-force. The Centre for Health Improvement (CHI), the NHS Performance Framework and the NHS Patient Survey will monitor the standards.

The first chapter of the book describes how a clinical governance culture incorporates effective clinical management and well-organised working conditions. Those working in primary care should be able to demonstrate that they are fit to practise as individual clinicians or managers (best practice in the management of coronary heart disease in this case), and that their working environment is fit to practise from. This section will be relevant to all readers, whether they are clinicians or primary care managers, so that they understand more of the context within which they work and how their individual contribution fits into the whole picture of healthcare.

Thereafter, each chapter of the book matches the topics in the National Service Framework for coronary heart disease[2] for England, to make it easier for practice teams and PCOs to address the expected standards of CHD care and services. We cover the evidence for the modern management of coronary heart disease. Sometimes we cite evidence from a review or compendium rather than the original literature, in order to simplify the text as far as possible.

The book culminates with simple examples of a personal development plan and a practice personal and professional development plan in Chapter 10.[3] Adopt a wide-based approach to improving quality – think of how you are establishing a clinical governance culture in your own practice team in your timed action plans. Make changes as a result – to your workplace, or to the equipment in your practice, or to the advice you give to patients, or to the way in which you manage and investigate coronary heart disease or complicating problems.

Try to use the opportunity of the National Service Framework for CHD to gain additional resources and invest effort in making your disease registers more effective, your data recording more consistent, and your preventive and management approaches more effective.

This book interfaces with another book in the series – Chambers R, Wakley G and Iqbal Z (2001) *Cardiovascular Disease Matters in Primary Care.* Radcliffe Medical Press, Oxford – which is written from a grassroots primary care perspective. That book includes chapters on the primary care management of stroke, hypertension, myocardial infarction, angina, heart failure and health promotion, including smoking cessation. Each chapter ends with a selection of reflective exercises for GPs, nurses and other primary care team members to complete. The completed reflective exercises build up to comprehensive personal development plans or practice personal and professional development plans. Some of the material is available online at: www.primarycareonline.co.uk.

Appendix 1 lists the main Read codes for classifying heart disease, and Appendix 2 contains useful comparative population data for a range of cardiac conditions. Appendix 3 includes a list of the standards, milestones and goals in the National Service Framework for Coronary Heart Disease for England, with the expected timetables. Finally, Appendix 4 lists details of useful sources of help.

CHAPTER 1

Clinical governance and the management of coronary heart disease

Clinical governance is about doing anything and everything required to maximise the quality of healthcare or services provided for, and received by, individual patients or the general population – in this case, those with coronary heart disease or who are at risk from it.[4,5]

We should be able to use clinical governance to improve the detection and control of chronic conditions such as coronary heart disease. Clinical governance is inclusive, making quality everyone's business, whether they are a doctor, a nurse or other health professional, a manager, a member of staff or a strategic planner. Good healthcare relies on the multidisciplinary team to support the person with coronary heart disease in self-managing their disease in as much as they are able to do so. Delivering best practice requires sufficient clinical staff who are up to date and relate well to their patients, working with efficient systems and patient-friendly procedures.

Components of clinical governance[5]

The components of clinical governance are not new. However, bringing them together under the banner of clinical governance and introducing more explicit accountability for performance is a new style of working.

The following 14 themes are core components of professional and service development which together form a comprehensive approach to providing high-quality healthcare services and clinical governance.[5] These are illustrated by the diagram shown in Figure 1.1.

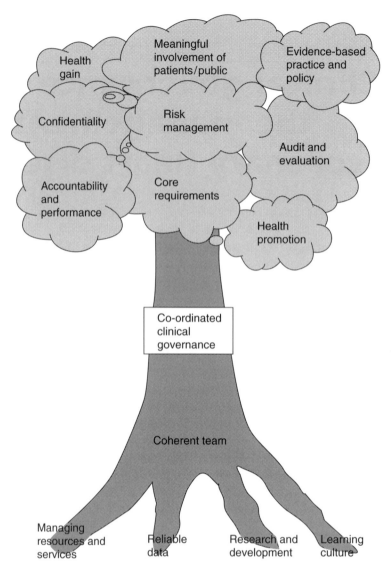

Figure 1.1: 'Routes' and branches of clinical governance.

If you interweave these 14 components into your individual and workplace-based personal and professional development plans, you will have addressed the requirements for clinical governance at the same time.[3,5]

1 *Learning culture*: for patients and staff in the practice or primary care organisation or working with public health experts or secondary care.

2   *Research and development culture*: in the practice or throughout the health service.
3   *Reliable and accurate data*: in the practice, across the primary care organisation and across the NHS as a seamless whole.
4   *Well-managed resources and services*: as individuals, as a practice, across the NHS and in conjunction with other organisations.
5   *Coherent team*: well-integrated teams within a practice, including attached staff.
6   *Meaningful involvement of patients and the public*: including those with coronary heart disease, those who care for them and the general population.
7   *Health gain*: from improving the health of staff and patients in a practice, between practices and in a primary care organisation.
8   *Confidentiality*: of information in consultations, in medical notes and between practitioners.
9   *Evidence-based practice and policy*: applying it in practice, in the district and across the NHS.
10 *Accountability and performance*: for standards, performance of individuals and the practice – both to the public and to those in authority.
11 *Core requirements*: good fit with skill mix and whether individuals are competent to do their jobs, communication, work-force numbers and morale at practice level.
12 *Health promotion*: for patients, the public, your staff and colleagues – both opportunistic and in general, or targeting those with most needs.
13 *Audit and evaluation*: for instance, of the extent to which individuals and practice teams adhere to best practice in clinical management.
14 *Risk management*: being competent to detect those at risk, and reducing risks and probabilities of ill health. This is really important in coronary heart disease.

The challenges to delivering clinical governance

Delivering high-quality healthcare with guaranteed minimum standards of care at all times is a major challenge. At present, the quality of healthcare is patchy and variable. We are not very good at detecting under-performance and rectifying it at an early stage. The small number of clinicians who do under-perform exert a disproportionately large effect on the public's confidence. Causes of under-performance in an individual might be a result of a lack of knowledge or skills, poor attitudes, ill health or a lack of resources. Poor management is nearly always a contributory reason for inadequate clinical services.

We need to understand why this variation exists and explore ways of reducing the inequalities. Variation in the quality of healthcare provided is common – between different practices in the same locality, between staff of the same discipline working in the same practice or unit, and in the care that is given to some groups of the population rather than others.

Clinical governance offers a co-ordinated approach to overcoming these areas of risk.[6] The complex cultural change that will be required to deliver uniformly excellent care is immense. We need to develop measurable outcomes that professionals, patients and the public consider to be relevant and meaningful. Then we can assess the progress made through implementing clinical governance in the milestones and goals set out in the National Service Framework (NSF) for coronary heart disease.

The Commission for Health Improvement (CHI)

CHI's definition of clinical governance for England and Wales is the framework through which NHS organisations and their staff are *accountable* for the quality of patient care. It covers the organisation's *systems and processes* for monitoring and *improving* services.[7]

CHI views clinical governance as having seven technical components:

- consultation and patient involvement
- clinical risk management
- clinical audit
- research and effectiveness
- use of information about the patient's experience
- staffing and staff management
- education, training, and continuing personal and professional development.

These seven technical components are matched by the following organisational components:

- organisational and clinical leadership
- direction and planning

- performance review
- patient and public partnership.

The Commission anticipates a four-year rolling programme, conducting clinical governance reviews in every NHS trust, and in health authorities with primary care groups in England, and in local health groups in Wales. CHI will also investigate serious service failures in the NHS.

Learning culture

Education and training programmes should be relevant to service needs, whether at organisational or individual levels. Continuing professional development (CPD) programmes need to meet both the learning needs of individual health professionals and the wider service development needs of the NHS. You should no longer opt for CPD activities according to what you *want* to do, but rather according to what you *need* to do. Clinical governance underpins professional and service development.

Box 1.1

Individual personal development plans
will feed into a
**workplace- or practice-based personal and
professional development plan**
that will feed into
the organisation's business plan
(the primary care organisation, the trust),
all of which are
underpinned by clinical governance.[3]

Multidisciplinary learning helps the team to work closely to provide well co-ordinated multidisciplinary care.

Applying research and development in practice

The findings of the many thousands of research papers about coronary heart disease that are published each year are rarely applied in practice. This is because few health professionals or managers read such journals regularly, so they are unaware of the research findings. Most practice teams do not have a system for reviewing important research papers and translating that review into practical action. The primary care organisation might help by feeding important new evidence to its constituent practices or the general public. Agreeing on local disease templates (e.g. for coronary heart disease) backed by resources should enable change to occur.

Box 1.2

Incorporating research-based evidence into everyday practice should promote policies on effective working, improve quality and contribute to a clinical governance culture.

Reliable and accurate data

Keep good written records of policies and audits that relate to coronary heart disease in the practice. An inspection at any time should show what audits have been undertaken and when, the changes in practice organisation that followed, the extent of staff training undertaken and the future programme of monitoring.

Well-managed resources and services

The things you need to achieve best practice should be in the right place at the right time and working correctly every time.

The primary care services to which the public requires access include information, advice, triage and treatment, continuity of care, personal care and other services. Systems should be designed to prevent and detect errors, so keep systems simple and sensible, and inform everyone how those systems operate so that they are less likely to bypass a system or make errors. Sort out good systems for the follow-up of patients with coronary heart disease, and for their clinical management.

Coherent teamwork

A team approach helps different team members to adopt an evidence-based approach to patient care – by having to justify their approach to the rest of the team.[8] The disciplines necessary for providing team-based coronary heart disease care include the GP and practice nurse, other community nurses, non-clinical staff, the dietitian and the community pharmacist, with help from other expert health professionals such as the cardiac specialist nurse, cardiac rehabilitation staff and hospital-based cardiologist.

Meaningful involvement of patients and the public

The aims of user involvement and public participation include better outcomes of individual care and better health of the population, more locally responsive services and greater ownership of health services.[9] Those planning the services should develop a better understanding of why and how local services need to be changed. For example, you might want to consult the public and health professionals about the closure of a community hospital, without which those with chronic conditions such as coronary heart disease may have to travel further for their care.

Health gain

The two general approaches to improving health are the 'population' approach, which focuses on measures to improve health throughout the community, and the 'high-risk' approach, which focuses on vulnerable individuals who are at high risk of the condition or hazard.

The population strategy aims to shift the whole distribution of a risk factor in a favourable direction.[10] However, the 'prevention paradox' means that preventive actions which greatly benefit the population at large may bring only small benefits for individuals. The high-risk approach aims to detect individuals who are at high risk of disease, and to lower their risk by treatment.

Box 1.3

Changing the population distribution of a risk factor is more effective than targeting people at high risk.[10]

Confidentiality

Confidentiality is a component of clinical governance that is often overlooked. The Caldicott Committee Report describes the following principles of good practice to safeguard confidentiality when information is being used for non-clinical purposes.[11]

- Justify the purpose.
- Do not use patient-identifiable information unless it is absolutely necessary to do so.
- Use the minimum necessary patient-identifiable information.
- Access to patient-identifiable information should be on a strict need-to-know basis.
- Everyone with access to patient-identifiable information should be aware of his or her responsibilities.

Evidence-based culture – policy and practice

There are several systems for grading evidence. A classification[12] that is often quoted gives the strength of evidence as shown in Box 1.4.

Box 1.4 Strength of evidence

Type 1: Strong evidence from at least one systematic review of multiple well-designed randomised controlled trials (RCTs).

Type II: Strong evidence from at least one properly designed randomised controlled trial of appropriate size.

Type III: Evidence from well-designed trials without randomisation, single group pre–post, cohort, time-series or matched case–control studies.

Type IV: Evidence from well-designed non-experimental studies from more than one centre or research group.

Type V: Opinions of respected authorities, based on clinical evidence, descriptive studies or reports of expert committees.

Other categories of evidence (*see* Box 1.5) are listed in the compendium of the best available evidence for effective healthcare, *Clinical Evidence*, which is updated every six months, and is perhaps more useful to the health professional in everyday work.[13]

Box 1.5

Beneficial:	Interventions whose effectiveness has been shown by clear evidence from controlled trials.
Likely to be beneficial:	Interventions for which effectiveness is less well established than for those listed under 'beneficial'.
Trade-off between benefits and harm:	Interventions for which clinicians and patients should weigh up the beneficial and harmful effects according to individual circumstances and priorities.
Unknown effectiveness:	Interventions for which there are currently insufficient data, or data of inadequate quality (this includes interventions that are widely accepted as beneficial, but which have never been formally tested in RCTs, often because RCTs would be regarded as unethical).
Unlikely to be beneficial:	Interventions for which lack of effectiveness is less well established than for those listed under 'likely to be ineffective or harmful'.
Likely to be ineffective or harmful:	Interventions whose ineffectiveness or harmfulness has been demonstrated by clear evidence.

The Scottish Intercollegiate Guidelines Network (SIGN) has produced over 50 evidence-based guidelines. It bases its recommendations on systematic reviews of the scientific literature. SIGN takes the view that guidelines do not provide answers to every clinical question, nor do they guarantee a successful outcome in all cases. Rather, the ultimate decision about a particular clinical procedure or treatment will depend on clinical judgement and each individual patient's condition, circumstances and preferences.[14] SIGN regards local ownership of the implementation of guidelines as crucial to success in changing practice. There are SIGN guidelines on *Lipids and the Primary Prevention of Coronary Heart Disease*[15] and *Secondary Prevention of Coronary Heart Disease Following Myocardial Infarction*.[16]

Accountability and performance

Clinicians may regard the performance assessment framework as a management tool that is not particularly relevant to their clinical practice. However, it does reinforce a clinical governance culture whereby there is a symbiotic relationship between good clinical and organisational management.

Box 1.6

The NHS performance assessment framework has six components, namely health improvement, fair access, efficiency, effective delivery of appropriate care, user/carer experience and health outcomes.

Health promotion

Smoking cessation services have been targeted at the 26 Health Action Zones in England and their disadvantaged populations. Most of them have concentrated on young people and pregnant women as priority groups to limit the harmful effects of smoking on future generations.[17]

Audit and evaluation

Audit will probably be the method you think of first for finding out how well you are doing and what it is you need to learn. You might look at the extent to which you are adhering to practice protocols – for instance, whether you are giving consistent advice to everyone with risks of coronary heart disease and/or diabetes about smoking habits, weight and exercise.[18]

Core requirements

The NHS Plan[19] describes the core requirements for the NHS in England which are part of a clinical governance culture in relation to the following:

- *partnership*: working together across the NHS to ensure the best possible care
- *performance*: acting to review and deliver higher standards of healthcare
- *the professions and wider work-force*: breaking down barriers between different disciplines – for instance, through multidisciplinary teamwork between GPs and nurses with pharmacists and other independent contractors
- *patient care*: access, convenient services, and empowerment to take full part in decision making about their own medical care and in planning and providing health services in general
- *prevention*: promoting healthy living across all sections of society, and tackling variations in care.

Risk management

Good practice means understanding and managing risk – both clinical and organisational aspects. Undertaking audit more systematically will reduce the risks of omission. Common areas of risk in providing healthcare services include the following:[6]

- out-of-date clinical practice
- lack of continuity of care
- poor communication
- mistakes in patient care
- patient complaints
- financial risk – insufficient resources
- reputation
- staff morale.

CHAPTER 2

Tackling coronary heart disease

Coronary heart disease (CHD) is the single commonest cause of death in the UK. CHD accounted for nearly one-quarter of all deaths in the UK in 1996 (28% of deaths in men and 18% of women).[20,21] Each year about 300 000 people have heart attacks in the UK, and only half of them survive. About 1.4 million individuals suffer from heart disease, including angina, and a high proportion of these are relatively young people.

Box 2.1 Facts about coronary heart disease[21]

- The premature death from CHD for South Asians living in the UK is 46% higher than the average for men and 51% higher for women.
- Coronary heart disease caused 150 000 deaths in the UK in 1996.
- The death rate from coronary heart disease in the UK is among the highest in the world. Only Ireland, Hungary and some eastern European countries have higher death rates.
- The decline in death rates from heart disease is slower among women than among men. Coronary heart disease death rates fell by 22% in women, compared with 27% in men, in England between 1983 and 1993.

It is estimated that 4% of all consultations in general practice are at least partly related to prevention and/or treatment of coronary heart disease. The cost to general practice of these consultations (excluding prescribing costs) was estimated to be £57.9 million for the UK in 1996.[21]

Coronary heart disease costs £10 billion per year to the UK economy. The majority of costs are social and are borne by employers, families and friends who care for those affected by coronary heart disease. The costs to the health service alone are £1.6 billion. A relatively small proportion (1%) of NHS expenditure is on cardiac prevention. The estimated cost of accident and emergency care for CHD is about £5 million.

An estimated £527 million is currently spent on drugs for CHD per annum. This could triple with increasing use of statins. A relatively small amount (£22 million) is spent on cardiac rehabilitation. The amount spent on community health and social care for coronary heart disease is difficult to estimate, but it may be of the order of £70 million.

One practice in South Yorkshire has shown what can be achieved by CHD prevention, as shown in Box 2.2.

Box 2.2 Risk assessment cuts admission rate

The winning entry in the coronary heart disease category of the Doctor Award competition for the year 2000 demonstrated how one practice cut admissions for myocardial infarction by 50%, so reducing secondary care costs by an estimated £28 000. The Barnsley practice had installed a computer offering a touch-screen risk assessment in the surgery waiting-room. The touch-screen computer can print out a patient's individual risk profile for them to discuss with the GP or nurse, showing the effects of their lifestyle on their own health.[22]

The National Service Framework (NSF) for coronary heart disease

The intended effect of the NSF is an overall improvement in the health of the population.

The NSF includes standards and milestones by which the quality of care and services can be monitored. It describes interventions that are known to be effective, and it recommends models of care to deliver those interventions. The NSF aims to provide the means to implement improved systems of care. Audit tools and performance indicators should help to ensure that services are of an acceptable minimum standard.

The NSF for coronary heart disease is based on 12 standards.[2] These standards were developed both to provide cost-effective care through improved services, and to reduce variations in service provision in primary and hospital care throughout England. Other countries in the UK are expected to follow suit.

The NHS Plan emphasised CHD priorities, namely specialist smoking clinics, rapid-access chest pain clinics, reduced 'call to needle' time for thrombolysis after heart attacks, systematic best practice, increasing capacity for revascularisation, and improved secondary prevention of coronary heart disease.[19]

Local delivery plans are being developed. Primary care organisations are leading on many aspects of these delivery plans based on local needs. Service plans and integrated programmes of individual care will be consistent with the evidence on effectiveness.

There are many variations in the quality and quantity of coronary heart disease services available across the UK. Rates of CHD vary according to social circumstances, gender and ethnicity. Differences across the social spectrum have been widening. Many people are not receiving or acting on advice and help that could stop them developing CHD in the first place. Moreover, many people with CHD are not receiving treatments of proven effectiveness. There are unjustifiable variations in quality and access to some CHD services, as the example in Box 2.3 shows.

Box 2.3 Many people with established cardiovascular disease do not receive lipid-lowering drugs[23,24]

The total cholesterol and lipid levels of more than 13 000 adults who were sampled from across England were measured. At least a quarter had adverse lipid profiles. The proportion of adults who were taking lipid-lowering drugs was 2.2%. Less than one-third of patients with a history of coronary heart disease or stroke had received lipid-lowering drugs. Recently recommended targets for cholesterol concentrations were reached by only one in ten patients who were eligible for treatment.

The NSF should result in the health service and other statutory agencies working together to improve the broader determinants of health, including housing, socio-economic inequalities and transport.

The priorities for the NSF are to enable:

- people who smoke to give up with help from smoking cessation clinics in their locality
- prompt help from the ambulance service for people with symptoms of a heart attack, so that they have a better chance of being resuscitated if they suffer a cardiac arrest
- people with a suspected heart attack to be assessed and treated with a

clot-dissolving drug within one hour of calling for medical help as appropriate
- people admitted to hospital with a heart attack to receive the most effective care, consistent with the best available evidence
- people with angina or heart failure to be assessed and managed according to the best available evidence
- people referred by their GP with suspected angina to be seen and assessed by a specialist within two weeks
- more facilities for coronary revascularisation, more cardiologists and more cardiac surgeons
- comprehensive programmes of rehabilitation and support for people who have had a heart attack, bypass surgery or angioplasty
- high-quality, compassionate care based on good symptom control, psychological support and open communication for people with uncontrollable symptoms of CHD, or who may be dying from CHD.

Work-force issues

Education and training, recruitment and retention of the current work-force will be key to implementing the enhanced and extended services. Work-force planning will need to anticipate the changes in skill mix and the additional numbers of staff required in primary and secondary care to reduce mortality and morbidity rates significantly.

Primary care

The changing NHS is making new demands on primary care, which require more general practitioners, primary care nurses, administration and management support staff. There is concern about where the extra nurses and doctors will be recruited from, and where the additional resources will be found to pay their salaries.

Some examples of the additional manpower, new skills and improvements in primary care infrastructure that are required include the following:

- establishment of disease registers – and monitoring of their accuracy and usage
- participation in the development and use of electronic protocols for the identification, prevention and management of coronary heart disease

- in-depth assessment of CHD and heart failure patients
- regular review of patients with CHD
- provision of specialist lifestyle change support services (e.g. smoking cessation clinics, exercise participation schemes)
- an increase in the number of people (e.g. with atrial fibrillation) who need to be anticoagulated
- application of clinical governance, education and audit
- cardiac rehabilitation programmes.

The primary care nurse's role will be enhanced by, for example, running secondary prevention clinics, specialist support clinics (e.g. smoking cessation clinics) and possibly heart failure clinics. They will need significant specialist knowledge and technical skills (e.g. interpretation of ECGs, knowledge of drugs, etc.).

General practitioners within a primary care organisation may choose to develop special interests in cardiology, which consequently take them away from core GP work.

Secondary care

The NSF standards place considerable demands on current secondary care cardiology services, particularly the 10-year goals for revascularisation. Pressures include the following:

- systems for rapid thrombolysis
- an increase in the number of investigations for acute myocardial infarction, angina, heart failure and surgery patients
- increased numbers of revascularisations
- setting up rapid-access chest pain and heart failure clinics
- an expansion of cardiac rehabilitation services.

There are significant manpower implications for cardiologists, specialist cardiac care and rehabilitation nurses, and cardiac technicians.

Primary prevention targeted at the population

Box 2.4 Standard 1 of the NSF

The NHS and partner agencies should develop, implement and monitor policies that reduce the prevalence of coronary risk factors in the population, and that reduce inequalities in the risks of developing heart disease.

The prevention of coronary heart disease is a national priority. The White Paper *Saving Lives: Our Healthier Nation* set targets to reduce the rate of coronary heart disease and stroke by 40% in those under 75 years of age by the year 2010.[1]

Box 2.5

Primary prevention is the range of treatments used in people without clinical evidence of cardiovascular disease.

Primary prevention of coronary heart disease can be instituted as a population approach. This is generally a long-term strategy which attempts to tackle the wider economic and social determinants of ill health.

We need to develop policies for reducing smoking, promoting healthy eating and physical activity, and reducing obesity that are targeted at the whole population. These policies and the associated interventions should be developed across primary care with those working in secondary care and other appropriate organisations – for instance, local authorities and the sports and leisure services – and education (in schools and further/higher education). Reducing the whole population's risk levels by just a small amount has more effect on overall morbidity and mortality than targeted approaches for high-risk individuals.[10]

Policies need to be pursued at national and local levels to improve the public health of communities and complement the clinical high-risk approach addressed through other standards.

There are a range of local plans and initiatives which can help with the prevention of coronary heart disease. These include the following:

- community development strategies
- Agenda 21/sustainable development/environmental strategies
- local transport plan
- Health Action Zones
- *Healthy Cities* and *UK Health For All*
- healthy living centres
- school health plans
- sport and leisure strategies
- regeneration initiatives (e.g. New Deal for communities).

All of these plans need the various partners to work together to operate them.

The main risk factors for coronary heart disease

These include the following.

Fixed factors

- Increasing age.
- Male sex.
- Family history (i.e. coronary heart disease before the age of 55 years in men and before the age of 65 years in women).
- Other vascular diseases (e.g. stroke).

Modifiable/lifestyle factors

- Smoking.
- Diet high in saturated fats.
- Diet low in fruit and vegetables.
- Excessive alcohol consumption.
- Physical inactivity.

Physiological/biological factors

- High total cholesterol and low-density lipoprotein.
- Raised blood pressure.
- Low plasma cholesterol and high-density lipoprotein.
- High plasma triglycerides.

- Diabetes.
- Obesity.
- Thrombogenic factors.

Box 2.6 Better health the more low-risk factors you have in your lifestyle[25]

'The big question, though, is whether combining all the different aspects of healthy living makes a substantial difference to health outcomes. If [you] were to give up smoking, stop drinking, lose weight, eat properly and take some exercise, would it make any difference?'

The answer from one study of 122 000 female nurses aged 30 to 55 years was that a low-risk-factor lifestyle reduces the likelihood of a heart attack or stroke by about 80% over 14 years or so.

Overweight and obesity

Being overweight is linked to raised blood pressure, raised blood cholesterol, low levels of physical activity and glucose intolerance/non-insulin-dependent diabetes.

About 45% of men and 34% of women in the UK are overweight (body mass index of 25–30) and an additional 16% of men and 18% of women are obese (body mass index of > 30).

Around 15% of boys and girls are overweight, while an additional 1.5% are obese.[21]

A sensible, balanced diet

Although there has been a long-term decline in the proportion of food energy derived from fat in the UK, the consumption of chocolate is increasing.

Scotland and Northern Ireland have a lower intake of fruit and vegetables compared with South-West and Eastern England. The average intake of vegetables and fruit in the UK is still only three portions a day, compared with the recommended intake of five portions a day. Total fruit and vegetable consumption in professional groups is at least 50% higher than that in unskilled manual groups.

Over 11 million children currently spend £2 billion of their own money on snacks and sweets. In one week the average 11-year-old eats:[21]

- three portions of chips
- four bags of crisps
- 42 biscuits
- six cans of soft drink
- seven puddings
- seven bars of chocolate.

Box 2.7

One piece of fruit is now being given free to 4- to 6-year-olds each day at school in line with the NHS Plan.[19]

Alcohol

In the UK, 28% of men and 13% of women consume more alcohol than is recommended (14 units per week for women and 21 units for men). Around 42% of young men (aged 16 to 24 years) and 27% of young women are estimated to be drinking more alcohol than the recommended limits. The proportion of women who drink more than the recommended amount is three times as high in the professional groups as it is in unskilled groups.[21]

Box 2.8 Proportion of coronary heart disease attributable to various modifiable risk factors in the USA[26]

	Estimated proportion (%)
Cholesterol level > 5 mmol/L	43
Physical inactivity	35
Cigarette smoking	22
Obesity	17

These figures give an indication of the relative importance of risk factors. However, the statistics will be different for the UK, as more of the local population are smokers and fewer are obese, compared with the USA.

Physical activity

Two out of three men (64%) and three out of four women (76%) lead a sedentary life. Only 31% of men and 20% of women are active enough to gain some protection against coronary heart disease.

By the age of 12 years, 16% of girls do not play sports out of school hours at all. By the age of 15 years, only 36% of girls engage in physical activity for at least 30 minutes on most days, compared with 71% of boys.[21]

Box 2.9 Promoting exercise in primary care[27]

One practice in Wales promotes physical activity through (i) Health Walks, (ii) Health Cycling and (iii) Green Gym.

Health Walks is a scheme that uses trained volunteers in the local community to lead walks on specific routes in the local area. Over 2000 walks involving 10% of the local population have been organised to date.

Health Cycling is a similar project involving organised cycle rides starting from the health centre, which take place in the summer.

The Green Gym provides alternative physical activity using graded exercise based on conservation work in the local community.

Contact: Sonning Common Health Centre, Practice Manager Tel: 0118 972 2188.

Diet and cholesterol

There have been many studies examining the individual dietary intake of saturated fats and cholesterol and the effect on cholesterol levels. The effectiveness of a low-fat diet depends on the extent to which a person adheres to advice, the content of the diet and the population studied (e.g. whether it is the general population or a population of individuals at high risk for coronary heart disease, in whom greater reductions have been demonstrated).

Studies of cholesterol-lowering interventions mediated by a population approach have shown only small changes in cholesterol, with the overall reduction being around 1–5%. Although such a reduction is almost insignificant for an individual patient, it is equivalent to a theoretical reduction of coronary heart disease mortality of up to 10% at a population level. In the UK this would be equivalent to avoiding 6000 deaths in people under the age of 75 years per year.

Blood lipids can be divided into different components, namely low-density-lipoprotein (LDL) cholesterol, high-density-lipoprotein (HDL) cholesterol and triglycerides. Low levels of HDL and high levels of LDL are associated with an increased risk of CHD. The ratio of total LDL cholesterol to HDL cholesterol is often used to assess the risk of CHD. In countries where the average cholesterol levels of the population are low, CHD rates tend to be low as well. The link between cholesterol level and future risk of CHD is continuous (i.e. there is no threshold above which CHD risks begin to increase). Thus lower levels of cholesterol are associated with a lower risk of CHD.

There is concern that low levels of blood cholesterol increase mortality from other causes, such as cancer, respiratory disease, liver disease and accidental/violent death, particularly following a pharmacological reduction in cholesterol levels. However, recent trials such as those involving HMG-CoA reductase inhibitors (statins) have not demonstrated any such relationship.[28] Increased mortality in individuals with low levels of cholesterol may be explained by the disproportionate number of people whose cholesterol levels have been reduced by a particular illness (e.g. cancer or a respiratory disease). The increased mortality is therefore thought to be due to pre-existing disease which is also causing the low cholesterol level.

Research has shown that garlic, oats and soya have a cholesterol-lowering effect. However, many of these research trials were small and of relatively short duration, and therefore they are difficult to interpret.

Smoking

Around 18% of deaths from coronary heart disease are due to smoking. Smoking in young people declined in the 1990s. About 23% of 15-year-olds smoked in 1999, compared with 30% in 1996.[29] One suggestion to explain the decline in smoking by young people is that increased ownership of mobile phones by young people absorbs their spare cash and may have partly replaced cigarettes as a boost to their personal image.

Box 2.10 Tobacco Control White Paper, *Smoking Kills*[30]

This White Paper provides a framework for local strategies which should aim to:

- reduce illegal sales of cigarettes
- monitor the advertising ban where it is introduced
- encourage media advocacy
- reduce smoking in public places
- work to support any national media campaign
- develop smoking cessation services.

Genetic factors

Single-gene disorders such as familial hypercholesterolaemia are particularly important because they may cause coronary heart disease at a young age. Genetic testing is complicated by ethical problems with regard to the commercial interest of insurance companies in predicting risk and weighting insurance premiums. Research into the genetic basis of coronary heart disease may lead to gene therapy.

Box 2.11 Summary of advice on healthy living for individuals[25]

1 Eat whole-grain foods (bread, rice or pasta) on four occasions a week.
2 Do not smoke, or else stop if you do. Nicotine patches, gum or inhaler might help a little. Try to reduce your smoking, as the more you smoke, the more likely you are to have either cancer or heart or respiratory disease. Therefore cut down to below five cigarettes a day and leave long portions of the day without a cigarette.
3 Eat at least five portions of vegetables and fruit a day, especially tomatoes (including ketchup) and red grapes, as well as salad all year round.
4 Consider using Benecol instead of butter or margarine. It does reduce cholesterol, and reducing cholesterol will reduce the risk of heart attack and stroke even in those whose cholesterol level is not particularly high. Reduce visible fat.
5 Drink alcohol regularly. The type of alcohol probably does not matter too much, but the equivalent of a couple of glasses of wine a day or a couple of beers is a good thing.
6 Eating fish once a week will not prevent you from having a heart attack in itself, but it reduces the likelihood of your dying from it by 50%.

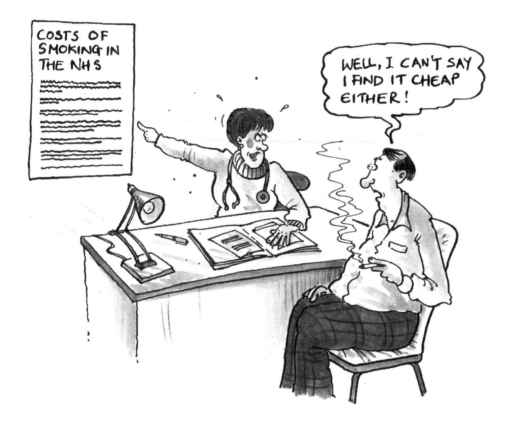

7 Take a multivitamin tablet every day, with at least 200 micrograms of folate. This can substantially reduce the likelihood of heart disease in some individuals.

8 Walking a mile a day, or taking reasonable exercise three times a week (enough to make you sweat or glow) will substantially reduce the risk of heart disease.

9 Your body mass index should be below 25. If you are overweight, lose the excess weight.

Targeting the more deprived communities

Much of the increased mortality in deprived communities is explained by the increased prevalence of risk factors. More than three times as many men of social class V smoke compared with those in social class I. There is a similar social class difference for obesity, vegetable and fruit consumption, and blood pressure – but not for the consumption of fat or for level of physical activity.[21] The death rate from coronary heart disease among unskilled men is three times higher than that among men of social class I (professionals).

Health Action Zone programmes are directed at deprived communities. They are often based on community development work which attempts to empower individuals and communities to take more responsibility for their own health and well-being. Local authorities and health authorities should work together increasingly to tackle the social determinants of health, and to implement anti-poverty strategies. When the general population is questioned about their perceived health needs and local solutions, they often prioritise issues such as community safety, although they recognise the adverse consequences of smoking and illicit drug use.

Implementing the National Service Framework for coronary heart disease is important

It will take more than the setting of standards and milestones to implement the NSF. Much will depend on good practice organisation, and the recording of data about individual patients in a consistent way across a practice, primary care organisation (PCO) or district in order to enable meaningful audit and forward planning. PCOs should anticipate work-force planning and training needs to be able to provide the improved and extended services envisaged by the NSF.

There are potentially immense benefits in reducing mortality and morbidity rates by ensuring uniformly effective care across all of the practices in the PCO's constituency. Clinical governance will underpin this work. Addressing the NSF should provide an opportunity to establish the infrastructure and culture of clinical governance across the primary care organisation, around a priority topic that will have knock-on benefits for other disease areas.

Similarly, developing clinical pathways both within primary care and with those working in secondary care will establish ways of working on coronary heart disease that can be used as a model for working on other disease areas.

Primary care organisations are expected to help to achieve the government's target to reduce the death rate from coronary heart disease and stroke in people under 75 years by two-fifths by 2010. This should include assessing local health needs, developing local strategies in partnership with other agencies and the health improvement programme, and priority setting within a finite budget. Identifying gaps in services and particularly gaps in funding should give PCOs the opportunity to address inequities in service provision, to secure additional resources and to tackle the root causes of deprivation with other local agencies.

Information and information technology (IT) will play a crucial role in meeting the NSF standards that are relevant to primary care, and should have a real impetus on the development of information/IT systems across the primary care organisation and beyond.

Roles and responsibilities of the primary healthcare team

These are just ideas, and are not meant to be comprehensive.

Primary care organisations

Primary care organisations can help to reduce heart disease in the population by:

- actively participating in local plans such as the health improvement programme (HImP). For instance, they might agree targets with other agencies for the reduction of coronary heart disease, and outline actions that primary care will undertake to achieve those targets
- supporting the involvement of local communities in the planning process, in particular engaging excluded groups of people
- participating in local multi-agency anti-poverty strategies. For example, the PCO could target primary care resources in areas of greatest need
- providing primary care information to profile local health needs and inequalities. For instance, the PCO could contribute practice-based information on immunisation rates, cervical cancer screening rates, etc.
- securing public health resources and expertise from health authorities, universities, and so on.

Primary healthcare teams

In general, primary healthcare team members are highly respected in the local community. They can endorse local strategies and plans and help to publicise them within the locality by, for example:

- local media campaigns to promote healthy nutrition
- writing to local schools to promote policies on healthy eating
- publicising and supporting various biking or walking initiatives in the local community (e.g. providing public support for walking to school (walking bus) initiatives through posters in the surgery, or suggesting this as patients consult)
- participating in exercise referral/prescription schemes.

GPs

GPs will need to provide leadership for the practice team. The investment in time and effort should pay off in terms of increased quality of care and services for patients, and more health gains.

GPs will need to ensure that:

- there are evidence-based practice protocols for all key aspects of CHD
- prescribing, primary/secondary prevention and management of CHD are in line with practice protocols
- the practice invests in staff learning new skills to support improved CHD services
- there is an equitable provision of care and services to all subgroups of the patient population.

Primary care nurses

Primary care nurses will have more opportunities to extend the range of their skills in managing secondary prevention of CHD (e.g. by running secondary prevention clinics).

In addition, nurses will need to be able to:

- manage CHD care through computerised templates and protocols
- undertake audits of the extent of adherence of patients, doctors, nurses and non-clinical staff to the practice's agreed evidence-based protocols
- give patients who are at risk of CHD, or those with established CHD, up-to-date information about their condition.

Pharmacists

Community pharmacists should be able to play a more substantial role in preventing and managing CHD than they have typically done in the past.

For example, they might:

- contribute to the assessment of risk status (over the counter, with near testing, information)
- contribute to supporting smoking cessation services (through supplying medication by prescription, advising customers, providing expert help about smoking cessation to individual smokers)
- work with local primary care teams on protocols and repeat prescribing (to improve the quality of care through multidisciplinary learning and working).

Patients

The more we know about the causes of CHD and ways of preventing and managing it, the more that patients who are at risk of CHD or who have established disease can do for themselves. For example, they can:

- adhere to recommended treatment
- follow sensible lifestyle advice
- support family members and friends who are at risk of CHD or who have established CHD.

Box 2.12 Tips for implementing the NSF for CHD from the primary care organisation's perspective

1 Implementing the NSF will require networking between and within a range of agencies (health and non-health). Avoid meeting overload by ensuring that clinicians and those with an interest in the wider population approaches are brought together only when there are areas of common interest. Check that:
   • the terms of reference, membership and tenure for any committee or working party have been agreed
   • everyone is included who needs to be a permanent member (can some people be co-opted for specific issues?)
   • the chair has appropriate skills and experience
   • the agendas of meetings are consulted upon and circulated well in advance
   • people are not dragged unnecessarily to all meetings, including those about issues that lie outside their knowledge or responsibility, just for the sake of agencies or partners being seen to work together in a high-profile way
   • decisions are made *at* meetings rather than outside them.
2 Before introducing IT systems, consider the IT implications of other national imperatives (e.g. other NSFs and the need for IT decision-making tools, etc.).
3 Invest in IT skills.
4 Invest in practice nurse time.
5 Establish a network between the local PCOs and the acute hospital trusts.
6 Adopt a project management approach at the PCO level. The NSF is complex, and PCOs will need to keep track of the progress of every practice towards various milestones and goals.
7 The PCO coronary heart disease leads should summarise the main points of the NSF and distribute and organise workshops to explain and explore local issues. Very few GPs and nurses are likely to read 250 pages of the NSF or other detailed national plans.
8 PCOs should consider the option of collaboration with the pharmaceutical industry, acute trusts or other organisations (commercial, educational, etc.) to help to facilitate implementation. Many PCOs have acquired additional funds for practice nurse time or an NSF co-ordinator through partnership with the pharmaceutical industry or acute trusts.

CHAPTER 3

Smoking cessation

Smoking is the single greatest cause of preventable illness and pre-mature death in the UK.[30-34] An estimated 13 million adults in the UK are smokers. Smoking rates have fallen steadily for the last two decades, except for the last two to three years, when rates have fluctuated. About 28% of adult men and 26% of adult women are currently smokers.

Appendix 2 includes statistics categorised by age and gender for the number of smokers you might expect in a typical practice of 10 000 patients.

Smoking is more common in lower socio-economic groups. Around 15% of men with professional jobs are smokers, compared with 45% of men in unskilled jobs. Smoking is more common in North-West England and in Scotland (31% and 30% of adults, respectively, compared with 24% of men who live in South-West England who are smokers).

Box 3.1 Standard 2 of the NSF

The NHS and partner agencies should contribute to a reduction in the prevalence of smoking in the local population.

More than 120 000 people die from smoking each year in the UK. This has been likened to the equivalent of a jumbo jet carrying more than 300 passengers crashing with no survivors – every day.

Smoking causes cancers, lung and heart disease, stroke, ulcers and peripheral vascular disease. Pregnant women who smoke are more likely to have low-birth-weight babies. Deaths that are caused by smoking include those due to cancer (30%), respiratory disease (34%), circulatory disease (15%) and digestive disease (9%).

Box 3.2 Smoking kills

Smoking kills around six times more people in the UK than road and other accidents, murders and manslaughter, suicide, poisoning, overdose and HIV added together.

The following diseases are caused in part by smoking (figures in parentheses are the percentages of all deaths from each disease that are estimated to be caused by smoking).

1 Cancer:
   • lung cancer (84%)
   • other respiratory cancers (66%)
   • oesophagus cancer (66%)
   • bladder cancer (38%)
   • kidney cancer (27%)
   • stomach cancer (25%)
   • pancreatic cancer (23%)
   • leukaemia (15%).
2 Respiratory disease:
   • chronic obstructive lung disease (83%)
   • pneumonia (16%).
3 Circulatory disease:
   • ischaemic heart disease (17%)
   • stroke (11%)
   • aortic aneurysm (15%).
4 Digestive disease:
   • ulcer of stomach and duodenum (44%).

Box 3.3

A total of 17 000 hospital admissions per year of children aged under five years are attributed to parents' smoking.[1] Passive smoking has been linked to asthma, glue ear and cot death in children.

Costs of smoking

The estimated annual cost of smoking to the NHS is £1.7 billion in terms of GP consultations, prescriptions and hospital care. For a typical health authority, that amounts to £14 million per year. At least seven in ten smokers visit their GP at least once each year. Smoking-related illnesses account for 8 million GP consultations in the UK annually.

The treatment of passive smoking-related illness in England and Wales costs around £410 million annually.

Smoking cessation

The benefits of smoking cessation are obvious. People who stop smoking before they reach middle age avoid most of their subsequent risk of lung cancer.

Every health authority in England has been set targets on the numbers of smokers who should receive specialist services and the numbers quitting smoking at the end of one year. In turn, primary care organisations have been set their own targets, and in some cases have agreed plans with their constituent general practices on their contribution towards meeting the national target.

Smoking cessation services have already been piloted in Health Action Zone (HAZ) areas, and more challenging smoking cessation targets have been set for them.

When they consult health professionals, smokers are not consistently warned of the dangers of smoking. About 29% of smokers who had seen GPs in the previous year had said that they had been given advice on smoking. In another survey, only 39% of pregnant women reported receiving advice about smoking.[35,36]

Brief advice from GPs for an average of three minutes may lead to only 2 or 3% of smokers stopping, and such poor success rates can be disheartening. However, if this was replicated in the whole population, the 2–3% of people quitting smoking would translate into thousands of smokers and enormous health benefits. It has been estimated that if GPs advised an additional 50% of smokers to stop smoking, this could translate into 75 000 extra ex-smokers a year in England alone.[37]

Common misconceptions about the cost-effectiveness of smoking cessation interventions include the beliefs that such services will increase healthcare spending, that smokers are too addicted to stop, and that local interventions will have little impact on overall population smoking cessation rates. However, enabling someone to stop smoking is one of the most cost-effective interventions a health professional can make.

Potential savings from smoking cessation for society include the gains for employers in terms of work attendance and productivity (due to improved health and fewer smoking breaks), a reduction in litter (i.e. cigarette butts) and a reduced risk of causing fires.

Services for smokers

Smoking cessation services should:[2]

- identify and record the smoking status of patients in general practice records
- provide advice on the various options for smoking cessation
- provide accurate information and advice on nicotine replacement therapy (NRT) and bupropion
- provide access to appropriate services, including intensive support through specialist services where this is required
- provide NRT for one week without charge to smokers who are entitled to free prescriptions
- urge smokers to persist in trying to give up
- provide access to the tobacco campaign helpline service (Tel: 0800 169 0169).

Intermediate-level smoking cessation services

These are defined as 'smoking cessation support based around general practice and can involve either one to one or group support led by a member of the primary care team, e.g. health visitor.'[2] This service can be shared between practices, and single-handed or smaller practices may wish to consider this option. The PCO or health authority may be able to provide resources (e.g. nurse time) to support this service.

Specialist smoking cessation clinics

Those smokers who require more intensive or specialist help should be referred to a specialist smoking cessation service.

A range of specialist smoking cessation clinics have been established throughout health authorities. The characteristics of specialist services are as follows.

- Smokers are offered support mainly in groups, but also on an individual basis if necessary.
- Support is offered by practitioners trained in smoking cessation techniques.
- Nicotine replacement therapy is offered, and is free for those not paying prescription charges.
- Success rates and, in particular, quit rates after one year are measured.

- Compliance is assessed by measuring carbon monoxide levels in expired air.
- A variety of self-help materials are also provided.

Success rates in smoking cessation

Around 10 million smokers in the UK have stopped smoking in the last 20 years. However, although two-thirds of smokers may want to stop, only 3% of smokers will succeed in their attempts to stop smoking if unaided, after a 12-month period.[35]

An early report on the smoking cessation services set up in Health Action Zones gives a rosy view of success rates (*see* Box 3.4 below). Obviously the confirmatory test will be to verify these self-reports and see whether such success is sustained after, say, one year.[17]

Box 3.4 Effectiveness of smoking cessation clinics

Twelve months after smoking cessation services were set up in Health Action Zones in England, around 14 600 people had set a 'quit date'. Four weeks later, 39% of those who had set a quit date reported that they had successfully quit smoking. Two-thirds of those who had set a quit date were entitled to free prescriptions and thus free nicotine replacement therapy.[17]

Table 3.1 An estimate of the relative effectiveness of various smoking interventions in the 'real world' rather than with highly motivated volunteers and staff[35]

Intervention	Percentage still abstinent after 12 months
Will-power alone	3
Self-help materials (e.g. audio tapes, videos, booklets)	4
Pharmacotherapy bought from a pharmacy	6
Smokers' clinic but no pharmacotherapy	10
Smokers' clinic plus pharmacotherapy	20

Group programmes seem to be more effective than self-help programmes. However, there is little evidence that group therapy is more effective than individual counselling of a similar intensity. The overall quit rate, including the background placebo quit rate in smokers' clinics, is estimated to be around 10%.

A combination of pharmacotherapy and motivational support has the best success rates.

Summary of effectiveness of interventions to help people to stop smoking[36]

- Advice from doctors, structured interventions from nurses, and individual and group counselling are effective.
- Generic self-help materials are no better than brief advice, but are more effective than doing nothing. Personalised materials are more effective than standard materials.
- All forms of nicotine replacement are effective.
- Bupropion and nortriptyline have been found to increase quit rates in a small number of trials.
- The usefulness of clonidine is limited by its side-effects.
- Anxiolytics and lobeline are ineffective.
- The effectiveness of aversion therapy, necamylamine, acupuncture, hypnotherapy and exercise is uncertain.

Pharmacotherapy for nicotine dependence

Nicotine addiction produces neurobiological changes in the brain. The World Health Organisation (WHO) classifies nicotine addiction as a disease.[35] Nicotine replacement therapy (NRT) weans the addicted smoker off nicotine by a controlled reduction in intake and a subsequent reduction in withdrawal symptoms. NRT is available in a range of forms, including the following:

- chewing gum
- transdermal patches
- nasal spray
- inhalers
- tablets.

All of the commercially available forms of NRT appear to be effective and increase quit rates by one and a half to twofold.

Abstinence from cigarette smoking is associated with a characteristic

Table 3.2 Nicotine withdrawal syndrome[37]

Symptom	Duration	Symptoms reduced by NRT*
Irritability/aggression	< 4 weeks	Yes
Depression	< 4 weeks	Yes
Anxiety	< 2 weeks	Yes
Restlessness	< 2 weeks	Yes
Poor concentration	< 1 week	Yes
Increased appetite	> 10 weeks	Yes
Urge to smoke	> 2 weeks	Yes
Night-time awakening	< 1 week	Not known
Decreased heart rate	> 10 weeks	Yes
Decreased adrenaline	< 2 weeks	Not known
Decreased cortisol	Not known	Not known

* NRT, nicotine replacement therapy.

set of signs and symptoms which may be labelled as nicotine withdrawal syndrome. Table 3.2 above illustrates which symptoms may be alleviated by nicotine replacement therapy.[37]

Bupropion

Bupropion seems to be more effective than nicotine replacement therapy in smoking cessation. Box 3.5 lists the indications for use. The evidence shows that:

> Oral bupropion is a non-nicotine preparation recently marketed as an aid to help stop smoking. It is available on the NHS as a prescription-only medicine. When used in a specialist setting and in conjunction with regular counselling, bupropion is at least twice as effective as placebo in helping patients to stop smoking. However, it is not clear what contribution the specialist setting makes to this outcome. Preliminary results suggest that bupropion is possibly more effective than a nicotine skin patch . . . but there are no published data on how bupropion compares with other forms of NRT.[38]

Insomnia and dry mouth are common. Bupropion is contraindicated in people who suffer from epilepsy, as it can cause seizures.

Box 3.5 Bupropion: indications for use

Bupropion is indicated for smokers if they:

- are motivated to quit
- have nicotine dependence
- have access to motivational support.

Indications of nicotine dependency include:

- smoking within 20 minutes of waking
- smoking regularly throughout the day
- smoking more than 15 cigarettes a day
- withdrawal symptoms on attempts to quit.

The safety and efficacy of bupropion have not been evaluated in people under the age of 18 years.

Acupuncture

Acupuncture is often promoted as a treatment for smoking cessation, and is believed to reduce withdrawal symptoms. However, there is no clear evidence that acupuncture is effective for smoking cessation.

Anxiolytics

Anxiety and symptoms of depression sometimes accompany nicotine withdrawal, and smoking cessation sometimes precipitates depression. However, there is little evidence that anxiolytics aid smoking cessation.

Hypnotherapy

Hypnotherapy is widely promoted to help smokers quit, in the belief that it acts on underlying impulses to weaken the desire to smoke or strengthen the will to stop. The evidence for the benefit of hypnotherapy is inconclusive. Uncontrolled trials claim to show benefit, but randomised controlled trials have not.[33]

Brief intervention

All clinical members of the primary care team should:

- ask about smoking at every opportunity
- advise all smokers to stop
- assist the smoker in stopping
- arrange follow-up.

Ask

Establish and validate the smoking status of all patients at every visit. Record the person's degree of interest in quitting smoking, but do not pressure patients who smoke to the extent that you make them feel bullied.

Advise

Explain the benefits to the patient of stopping smoking, and the risks of continued smoking. Personalise this message.

Assist

Tips for increasing the likelihood of someone stopping smoking include the following.

- Set a date for stopping. Ideally the patient should quit smoking altogether on that day.
- Explore what has helped and hindered when the patient has tried to stop before.
- Establish what will be the likely problems in the future and what would help to resolve these.
- Enlist the help of family and friends.
- Consider other issues such as the use of alcohol and how that might sap their will-power.
- Discuss how to avoid putting on weight as a consequence of stopping smoking.
- Consider using NRT or bupirone.

Figure 3.1 shows the cycle through which a smoker might progress before quitting. You will need to refine your approach depending on whether the smoker is still contemplating whether to make the change or is actually preparing to change (i.e. give up smoking). They may need help in maintaining the change if they are not to relapse and start smoking again.

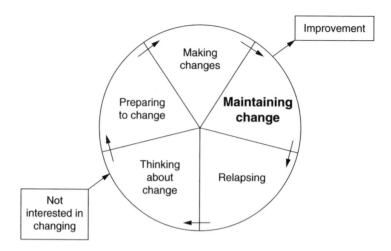

Figure 3.1: The process of change.

Establish smoking cessation services in your practice as laid out in Figure 3.2, using the information about the roles and responsibilities of the primary care team on the following pages.

Roles and responsibilities of the primary healthcare team

These are just ideas and are not intended to be comprehensive.

Primary care teams

Primary care teams need to decide how the various responsibilities for smoking cessation can be allocated.

- Agree on a lead/champion for smoking issues.
- Plan the training needs of individuals according to their roles and responsibilities in the overall smoking cessation programme.
- Set up an intermediate-level smoking cessation service.
- Agree on a protocol for referral into both the intermediate and specialist smoking cessation services.
- Collect data about the numbers of patients receiving services and outcomes in terms of smoking cessation quit rates.
- Target high-risk patients (e.g. those with diabetes) for quit-smoking interventions.

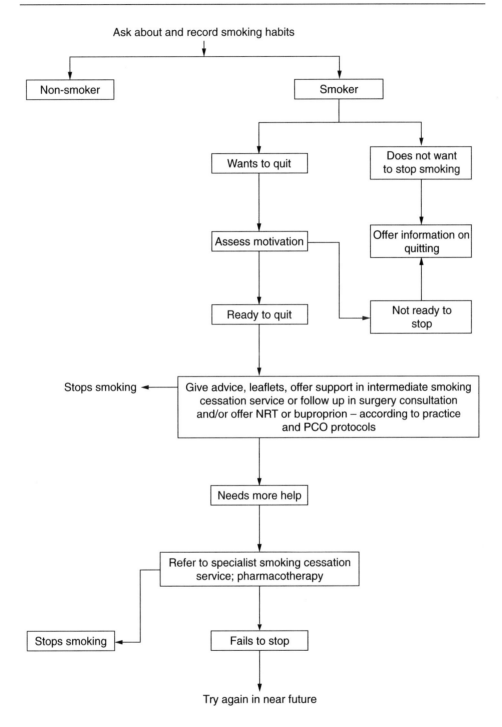

Figure 3.2: Smoking cessation – protocol for intervention by GP or community nurse (modified from Fowler, 2000[39]).

GPs

- Oversee the development of a practice-based smoking cessation service.
- Draft or agree a primary care team protocol for practice-based smoking cessation services.
- Ensure that smoking status is recorded in the patient records.
- Attempt to deliver brief intervention to all smokers.
- Try to stay motivated to urge smokers to quit.
- Find out 'what you do not know you do not know' and how you might rectify that in your personal development plan.
- Prescribe appropriate drugs for smoking cessation.

Primary care nurses (practice and district nurses, health visitor, midwife)

- Keep motivated to urge smokers to quit.
- Contribute to the drafting of a practice protocol for smoking cessation.
- Identify your own training needs and present them to your GP or practice manager.
- Deliver practice-based smoking cessation support (e.g. one-to-one or group-based support via a nurse-run clinic).
- Ask, advise, assist and urge smokers of all patient groups to quit.

Practice managers

- Secure resources from the PCO or health authority for an intermediate practice-based smoking cessation service (e.g. nurse time, smoking cessation support materials such as posters, smokelysers, health promotion leaflets, expertise on health promotion).
- Facilitate the assessment and meeting of staff training needs.
- Make arrangements for data collection to monitor performance and adherence to practice protocols.
- Develop a marketing strategy for promoting local smoking cessation services to patients.

CHAPTER 4

Secondary prevention of coronary heart disease

The National Service Framework (NSF) requires us to apply the secondary prevention measures of Standard 3 before tackling the primary prevention programme of Standard 4 (*see* Chapter 5).

Box 4.1 Standard 3 of the NSF

General practitioners and primary care teams should identify all people with established cardiovascular disease and offer them comprehensive advice and appropriate treatment to reduce their risks.

Secondary prevention aims to prevent the progression of coronary heart disease in individuals with existing vascular disease.[13–16,40–42] It is aimed at those people who already have heart disease such as angina, myocardial infarction, or who have undergone revascularisation by angioplasty or coronary artery bypass grafting (CABG). Patients with cardiovascular disease such as transient ischaemic attacks (TIAs), stroke and peripheral vascular disease should also be included.

A range of therapeutic and non-therapeutic interventions can substantially reduce the risks for those with coronary heart disease – by up to 60%.[13] These interventions can slow and perhaps even reverse the progression of established coronary heart disease.

If patients with coronary heart disease modify their risk factors, the rate of progression of their atherosclerosis and the risk of further cardiac events decreases proportionately. Patients who have already suffered a myocardial infarction have a threefold risk of suffering from another ischaemic event. The risk of death following a myocardial infarction is increased by 20 times over a 10-year period, compared with the risk for men with no signs of cardiovascular disease.

There are substantial variations in the uptake of these interventions across the UK, and enormous variations in the quality of care between practices. National audits in primary and secondary care have suggested that a relatively small proportion of those who could benefit are receiving all of the appropriate advice and treatment. The patients with the greatest need are often receiving poorer care.

Identifying and treating those at greatest risk of coronary events is one of the highest priorities for the NSF. Treatment of this group of people is also very cost-effective. A relatively small number of people need to be treated to prevent a cardiac event, as Table 4.1 shows.

The NSF for CHD recommends that patients who have had a stroke are also included on the secondary prevention register. The management of stroke patients is beyond the remit of this book. You can read more about managing stroke in: Chambers R, Wakley G and Iqbal Z (2001) *Cardiovascular Disease Matters in Primary Care*. Radcliffe Medical Press, Oxford.

Secondary prevention for patients with coronary heart disease within the primary care setting covers a range of therapeutic and non-therapeutic measures. Each individual patient needs a baseline assessment and management plan.

Many patients with coronary heart disease are elderly and have a range of additional problems such as arthritis and chronic obstructive airways disease. Uptake of all of the effective interventions could lead to a considerable increase in the numbers of drugs for individual patients (i.e. there is a danger of polypharmacy and drug interactions).

The aims of secondary prevention in modifying risk factors are often long term, and lifestyle changes in particular are notoriously difficult to achieve.

What patients should expect

Patients who have coronary heart disease should be offered a comprehensive assessment of their condition within their practice. They should receive a full explanation and participate in deciding on an individually tailored management plan based on the best available evidence. The programme of care should include effective interventions for secondary prevention.

There should be sufficient resources for convenient:

- access to specialist support (e.g. specialist smoking clinics, dietary interventions, exercise programmes, specialist rehabilitation support)
- referral to cardiologists for cardiac angiography and other investigations, etc.

Table 4.1: Comparison of the treatment benefits from interventions to prevent cardiovascular events (adapted from Sivers, 1999[40])

Problem and therapy	Events prevented	Estimated number of patients who need to be treated for five years to prevent one event (NNT)
Medication for severe hypertension (diastolic blood pressure 115–129 mmHg)	Death, stroke or myocardial infarction	3
Coronary artery bypass graft for left mainstem disease	Death	6
Aspirin for transient ischaemic attack	Death or stroke	6
HMG-CoA reductase inhibitor (simvastatin) post-myocardial infarction	Death, coronary event or coronary artery bypass graft/PTCA* or stroke	6
Warfarin for atrial fibrillation	Stroke	7
Angiotensin-converting-enzyme (ACE) inhibitor for left ventricular dysfunction post-myocardial infarction	Cardiovascular death or hospitalisation for chronic heart failure	10
Aspirin post-myocardial infarction	Cardiovascular death, stroke or myocardial infarction	12
Beta-blocker post-myocardial infarction	Death	21
ACE inhibitor for left ventricular dysfunction	Cardiovascular death or hospitalisation for chronic heart failure	21
HMG-CoA reductase inhibitor for primary prevention	Death, coronary event or coronary artery bypass graft/PTCA* or stroke	26
Medication for mild hypertension (diastolic blood pressure 90–109 mmHg)	Death, stroke or myocardial infarction	141

* PTCA, percutaneous transluminal coronary angioplasty.

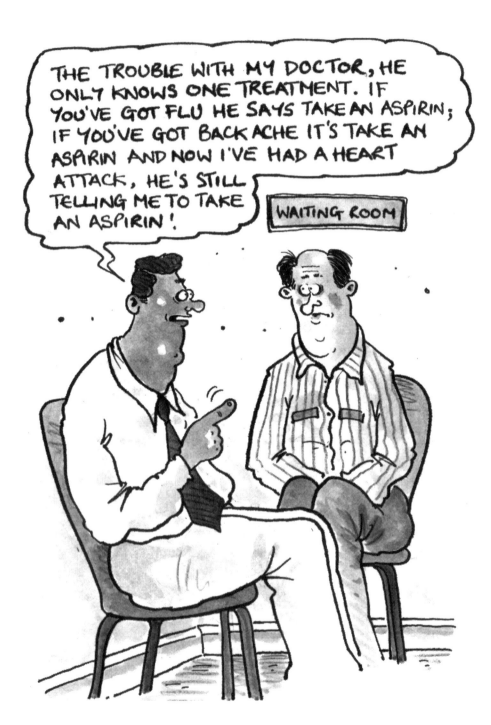

Arrangements for follow-up and review of coronary heart disease should be similar to other chronic disease management programmes, such as those for diabetes and asthma.

Non-pharmacological measures

Smoking

Studies suggest that individuals with coronary heart disease will reduce their risk of further fatal and non-fatal events by up to 50% over two years by giving up smoking. Those who continue to smoke are at up to three times higher risk of death compared with those who have stopped.

Smoking also reduces the prevalence of angina following a heart attack. Patients with angina who continue to smoke double the risk of subsequent cardiac events.[40]

Cholesterol lowering by diet

People who have recently had a myocardial infarction are more likely to be motivated to follow strict diets. However, research has not found any significant change in the overall coronary heart disease mortality following dietary interventions alone in high-risk patients. One explanation for this might be that dietary interventions often substitute total fat or carbohydrate, which reduces the levels of HDL cholesterol as well as LDL cholesterol. If the LDL/HDL ratio is unaffected, the magnitude of the coronary heart disease risk will also be unaffected. Therefore it is important to lower CHD risk, rather than focusing solely on a reduction in the cholesterol level.

Oily fish and Mediterranean diet

Increased intake of oily fish and a trial of a Mediterranean diet have both been shown to reduce CHD mortality after a heart attack without affecting cholesterol levels. The use of these interventions among people in the general population or at lower risk of CHD has not been tested.[13]

Obesity

No trials have been undertaken to assess the effect of weight reduction in secondary prevention, and therefore it is not known whether obesity is an independent risk factor. However, weight reduction should become part of secondary prevention management plans because of the adverse effect of obesity on other risk factors.[40]

Alcohol

The British Heart Foundation recommends that alcohol consumed in moderation may be beneficial for patients with established heart disease. However, higher alcohol intake at the population level has enormous adverse social and health consequences.

Cardiac exercise rehabilitation

Cardiac exercise rehabilitation following myocardial infarction has been shown to reduce all causes of mortality by 24%.[13] All patients with heart disease who have no contraindications to exercise should take regular aerobic exercise at least three times a week for 20–30 minutes.

Pharmacological interventions

Antiplatelet therapy[13,43]

Antiplatelet therapy reduces the risk of:

- vascular death by one-sixth
- non-fatal myocardial infarction by one-third
- non-fatal stroke by one-third

when used for secondary prevention of myocardial infarction, regardless of age, gender, diabetes or hypertension.

   Aspirin is associated with an overall reduction in myocardial infarction, stroke or vascular death of 25%. Different aspirin dose regimens have similar benefits.

Low-dosage aspirin (75 mg per day) reduces cardiovascular risk in well-controlled hypertensive patients who have cardiovascular complications.

Beta-blocker drugs

Beta-blocker treatment reduces total mortality, sudden death and reinfarction rates following myocardial infarction. The beneficial effects last as long as the treatment continues. The benefits of long-term beta-blockade result in a 20% reduction in risk of death, a 25% reduction in risk of reinfarction and a 30% reduction in risk of sudden death.

Statins[13,44,45]

Statins constitute the single most effective type of treatment for reducing cholesterol levels and reducing cardiovascular risk. There is a depression of lipids following a myocardial infarction which can last for an average of six weeks. It is therefore essential to measure the lipid profile 6–12 weeks after an acute myocardial infarction. If it is below the threshold at the time of an event, repeat the measurement in 6–12 weeks.

The Scandinavian Simvastatin Survival Study (4S) randomised patients who had had a myocardial infarction, or who had angina with a positive exercise test.[44] The intervention group received simvastatin, and the mean cholesterol reduction after five years was 28%. The total mortality was reduced by 30%, and there was a 42% reduction in deaths due to coronary heart disease. The need for coronary artery surgery or angioplasty was also reduced. The LIPID study of long-term intervention with pravastatin in ischaemic disease confirmed and extended the findings of the 4S study in a larger series of patients.[45]

The Cholesterol and Recurrent Events (CARE) study[46] using pravastatin showed that even treating patients with average cholesterol levels (6.2 mmol/L) produced a reduction in cholesterol, which was associated with reductions in CHD events and mortality. However, the overall mortality was not significantly reduced.

Statins appear to provide benefits in addition to those that result from the use of other secondary prevention interventions, such as aspirin and beta-blocker drugs.

Lipid-lowering therapy is covered in detail in Chapter 5 on primary prevention.

ACE inhibitors [13,47]

Angiotensin-converting-enzyme (ACE) inhibitor drugs improve asymptomatic left ventricular dysfunction following myocardial infarction.

Patients with clinical evidence of heart failure following myocardial infarction showed a 27% reduction in the risk of death and a 19% reduction in vascular events following treatment with ACE inhibitors.

Box 4.2 ACE inhibitors and the HOPE trial[47]

This study of more than 9000 high-risk patients aged 55 years or over with vascular disease or diabetes plus one other cardiovascular risk factor found that there was a reduction in myocardial infarction, stroke or death from cardiovascular causes when ramipril was compared with placebo treatment. Patients with heart failure were excluded from the trial.

There were significantly fewer diabetic complications (diabetic nephropathy and diabetic retinopathy) among patients with diabetes who took ramipril. The beneficial effects could not be attributed to a reduction in blood pressure alone, as the overall observed blood pressure reduction was only 2–3 mmHg.

The HOPE study (*see* Box 4.2) has now extended the evidence base for ACE inhibitors. The study suggests that ACE inhibitors have a preventative role in patients who are at high risk of cardiovascular disease. An estimated 80% of diabetic patients in primary care would qualify for an ACE inhibitor if the conclusions from the HOPE study were followed through.

Although the NSF for coronary heart disease promotes secondary prevention registers within primary care and comprehensive packages of preventative measures for patients with CHD, it does not refer to the HOPE study. Most patients on CHD registers will have an additional risk factor and would therefore qualify for an ACE inhibitor if the findings of the HOPE study were implemented. For instance, it has been calculated that up to 25% of the population over the age of 54 years would be eligible for treatment with ACE therapy.[47]

Use of anticoagulants[13]

There is some evidence that anticoagulant therapy reduces the risk of reinfarction and cerebrovascular events. However, the routine use of anticoagulants is not indicated, but anticoagulants are commonly used for large anterior myocardial infarcts and in patients with left ventricular aneurysms.

Anti-arrhythmic agents[13]

The evidence for the benefits of anti-arrhythmic agents following a myocardial infarction in terms of a reduction in mortality are unclear, and further research is needed.

Achieving optimal blood pressure control[48]

In general, the optimal target blood pressure is below 140/85 mmHg. Low levels of diastolic blood pressure provide protection against cardiovascular events and stroke in patients with ischaemic heart disease. A diastolic blood pressure of 80 mmHg provides protection against major cardiovascular events and mortality in a person with diabetes, and highlights the importance of tight blood pressure control in individuals with type 2 diabetes. The risk of systolic hypertension is as great if not greater than that of diastolic hypertension.

The presence of hypertension does not contraindicate the use of antiplatelet therapy. Aspirin is beneficial in patients with heart disease and hypertension, as well as in those with other high-risk factors, such as diabetes. However, as the benefits of treating younger hypertensive patients with aspirin are likely to be smaller, the risk of bleeding from a stomach ulcer assumes a greater importance, and therefore the use of aspirin cannot be justified routinely.

The British Hypertension Society guidelines[49] recommend 75 mg of aspirin for hypertensive patients over 50 years of age who have good blood pressure control and either target organ damage or diabetes.

Box 4.3

The use of aspirin routinely for hypertension in patients at low risk is not justified at present.

Myocardial infarction is covered in more detail in Chapter 6.

Comparison of current practice with Standard 3 of the NSF

There is considerable potential to improve secondary care prevention in the UK. The example in Box 4.4 below illustrates this.

Box 4.4 Action on secondary prevention through intervention to reduce events[50]

An audit of 2500 patients drawn from 12 specialist cardiac centres and 12 general hospitals assessed whether major coronary risk factors (cigarette smoking, obesity, hypertension, hyperlipidaemia, diabetes and family history) and the management of these factors were recorded in patients' notes. The audit also assessed changes in their risk factors and whether family members had been given the appropriate advice about CHD risk factors, and it described their management six months after hospital admission. All of the patients in this audit study had either had a heart attack or undergone a revascularisation procedure.

The results showed that risk factor recording was patchy. Around 60% of patients had no record of their lipid levels, and 25% did not have their family history recorded. At the six-month assessment, 20% of patients were smoking, 75% of patients were overweight, up to 25% of patients remained hypertensive, and 75% of patients had cholesterol levels higher than 5.2 mmol/L. One-third of the patients were taking beta-blocker drugs, and one-fifth were not taking aspirin at follow-up.

(This study was undertaken when the evidence for lipid reduction was being established and disseminated. This may partly explain the poor management of lipids described here.)

In another study of around 2000 patients on existing coronary heart disease registers in general practices in Scotland, researchers found considerable potential to increase secondary prevention in primary care. Only 63% of these patients were taking aspirin, 32% were taking beta-blocker drugs and 40% of those with heart failure were taking angiotensin-converting-enzyme (ACE) inhibitors. Hypertension management was consistent with current guidelines for 82% of patients, but only 17% of patients had evidence-based management of hyperlipidaemia. Just over half (51%) of them took little or no exercise,

18% were smokers, 64% were overweight and 52% ate more fat than was recommended. For virtually all of the patients at least one aspect of their medical management was suboptimal, and for about half of them at least two aspects were suboptimal. Similarly, nearly all patients had at least one high-risk behaviour and nearly two-thirds of them had at least two such behaviours. This study also confirms the considerable opportunity that exists for improving secondary prevention of coronary heart disease in general practice.[51]

Box 4.5 Healthy start programme/primary prevention of CHD[27]

A practice in Northumberland has a multidisciplinary approach to targeting all at-risk patients and introducing a systematic approach to care. Patients at risk as well as those with existing CHD are identified and invited to a nurse-led clinic with doctor input, to consider all aspects of prevention, investigation and management.

Contact: The Marine Medical Practice. Tel: 01670 396520.

Developing a structured approach to the management of secondary prevention of coronary heart disease

1 Agree a practice plan for implementing Standard 3 of the NSF.
2 Create a disease register of all people with coronary heart disease within the practice.
3 Develop a coronary heart disease secondary prevention service which offers a programme of care to all patients with coronary heart disease.
4 Develop a protocol.
5 Evaluate progress.
6 Involve patients with coronary heart disease or their carers in giving you feedback about their experiences, and in planning and monitoring services and care.

1 Agree a practice plan

Consider a range of factors such as national priorities, the PCO's priorities, local issues and local interests. Undertake local audits, and review cost pressures and workload pressures, etc.

Reach a common understanding within the primary care team of national issues, the issues within the practice and the evidence for effective interventions. Check that the primary care team accepts the evidence and agrees on everyone's roles and responsibilities.

The plan will require:

- consensus among doctors, nurses and support staff
- appropriate information systems
- access to evidence and skills to interpret that evidence
- understanding of the financial implications, particularly the prescribing of statins.

2 Creating a register

Registers can be used either for planning purposes or to help with the management of disease. A disease register is needed to implement Standard 3 by:

- helping to identify all of the patients with coronary heart disease
- facilitating baseline assessment of patients
- providing a recall system to review patients at agreed intervals
- facilitating a structured evidence-based approach to management
- helping to demonstrate change in processes or outcomes of care via audit.

The following steps need to be taken to develop the register.

1 Agree the definitions (e.g. who to include or exclude, age, diagnoses), including the Read codes (*see* Appendix 1 for examples).
2 Identify patients by searching for those who meet Read-code definitions. This could be done through a variety of mechanisms, including the following.
   - Search GP computer records for patients receiving certain drugs (e.g. glyceryl trinitrate, nitrates, calcium-channel blockers and statins) initially. Drug groups such as ACE inhibitors will pick up hypertensive patients, too.
   - Identify patients who are known to the primary care team.
   - Ask hospitals for a list of patients who have been discharged during the last few years.
   - Ask the general patient population to come forward via publicity (e.g. newspaper articles and posters in the surgery). This can dramatically increase the numbers of patients who are identified.
3 Validation.
   - Check that the patients with CHD who have been identified meet the agreed criteria. The practice nurse might validate those

with a clear diagnosis and leave the remainder for the GP to assess by examining individual patients' notes. This process will be time-consuming!

- Check whether the numbers of patients identified are broadly similar to the numbers expected (*see* Appendix 2 for figures from a typical patient population of 10 000).

4   Enter the patient data on the computer. The data need to be summarised using a template.

5   Use the register to call patients for review and to follow up patients.

6   Find a method (manual or electronic) for tagging a patient's medical records once they have been checked.

7   Link to decision-making tools such as Prodigy. Ideally a tool to measure CHD risk should also be available (*see* Chapter 5 on primary prevention).

8   Maintain an accurate and up-to-date register when:
- summarising patient records
- entering new patients who join the practice, are discharged from the hospital as out- or in-patients with a diagnosis of coronary heart disease, or are diagnosed with CHD within the practice
- removing patients who leave the practice or die
- searching the database for patients who have not been assessed or who have been reviewed within the agreed timeframe.

9   Use information in registers to audit and evaluate performance.

10   Revisit the practice plan and re-audit.

Box 4.6 Using the general practice health promotion scheme to establish secondary prevention registers

It has been found that 95 out of 98 practices in South Staffordshire Health Authority established CHD secondary prevention registers before the NSF was launched in the year 2000. Currently, most practices are providing structured care through either nurse-led clinics or GP-based care. This was achieved by:

1   linking the development of registers with payments related to the general practice health promotion scheme

2   devolving the administration of the practice health promotion scheme to localities (which preceded PCOs) and then primary care groups when they were created

3   providing incentive payments to practices for identifying patients who would benefit from aspirin and providing audit data (a local initiative entitled *The Aspirin Project*).

3 Develop a coronary heart disease secondary prevention service which offers a programme of care to all patients with coronary heart disease

Secondary prevention clinics provide an opportunity for structured care through a full assessment of the patients' needs and provision of a comprehensive package of interventions. Explore the variations of a nurse-led clinic (*see* Box 4.7 below and the examples that follow in this chapter).

Box 4.7 A nurse-led secondary prevention clinic in Preston[27]

A practice in Preston has a nurse-led clinic offering secondary prevention of CHD. A manual has been produced which covers the following:

- creation and maintenance of a practice register
- suggested audit activity and benchmarks
- protocols for patient assessment
- management of clinical and lifestyle factors
- medication review
- systems assessment
- investigations
- templates of letters and assessment records.

Contact: Lytham Road Surgery. Tel: 01772 716033.

---

4 Develop a protocol

Develop an evidence-based protocol and methods for recording patient data via a template (ideally an electronic version). This needs to be evidence based and consistent with local and national guidelines. Do not reinvent the wheel. Adapt existing guidelines for local circumstances (*see* Box 4.8 and the example of a protocol for a nurse-led secondary prevention clinic on pages 61 to 65).

Box 4.8 The interventions that patients with diagnosed CHD or other occlusive arterial disease should receive unless contraindicated

- Advice about how to stop smoking.
- Information about other modifiable risk factors, and personalised advice about how they can be reduced.

- Advice and treatment to maintain blood pressure below 140/85 mmHg.
- Low-dose aspirin (75 mg daily), or clopidogrel if aspirin is contraindicated.
- Statins and dietary advice to lower serum cholesterol concentrations to less than 5 mmol/L.
- ACE inhibitor drugs for patients who have left ventricular dysfunction, and for a wider group of patients if the findings of the HOPE study are implemented.
- Beta-blocker drugs for patients who have had a myocardial infarction, and for first-line prophylaxis for angina.
- Warfarin or aspirin for patients aged over 60 years who also have atrial fibrillation.
- Meticulous control of blood pressure and glucose in patients who also have diabetes.

Secondary prevention clinics

You might opt for:

- nurse-led clinics
- GP clinics
- opportunistic reviews by GPs and other members of the primary care team.

Secondary prevention clinics run by nurses in general practice may improve the uptake of secondary prevention measures within primary care, as the example in Box 4.9 illustrates.

Box 4.9 The effectiveness of nurse-led secondary prevention clinics

A study of 1200 patients in 19 general practices in Scotland examined the effectiveness of secondary prevention clinics compared with normal routine care. Patients with coronary heart disease who were aged 80 years or less were studied. Half of the patients in the study were invited to a secondary prevention clinic within their practice, run by nurses who assessed their symptoms, treatment and lifestyle factors in a structured way.

They were compared with the others who received normal care from their general practitioners. The clinics ran for one year.

Patients were followed-up every two to six months. General health was assessed using the Short Form 36 (SF36) scale, and mental health was assessed using the Hospital Anxiety and Depression Scale.

There were significant improvements in the health status of patients who attended the secondary prevention clinics, and a reduction in reported worsening of chest pain. However, there was no significant effect on anxiety or depression. The authors concluded that secondary prevention clinics lead to improvements in patients' health status as well as reducing hospital admissions.[52]

Box 4.10

One GP has commented: 'Since running a nurse-led secondary prevention clinic for two years, we have found that many patients have reported an improvement in their quality of life and particular improvements in angina symptoms'.

---

5 *Evaluation*

Evaluate progress against the milestones in the NSF for CHD.[2] At practice level, this will mean that clinical teams meet at least once every three months to plan and discuss clinical audit, that medical records are well organised, and that there is a systematically developed and maintained practice-based CHD register in place. Appendix 3 lists the milestones in more detail. Detailed audit criteria against which primary care will be assessed can be found in the CHD NSF documents.[2]

The performance of primary care organisations and health authorities in delivering health services in general may be judged by the NHS Performance Assessment Framework (*see* Chapter 1).

6 *Patient participation*

Feedback from patients is very valuable when honing services to be more convenient and accessible to different patient groups. You might ask patients directly how your services could be improved – for example, by means of a short questionnaire attached to repeat prescriptions, administered by the district nurse to housebound patients, or given to patients attending smoking cessation clinics for instance.

Develop a system for collecting patients' comments, rather than waiting for the occasional patient complaint. Look for patterns, and see whether you can anticipate problems by responding to negative comments.

Nurse time for secondary prevention clinics

Much of this work is over and above what general practices will have been doing in a systematic way. Therefore the additional work will require extra resources. Practices will need to plan how much time to allocate to secondary prevention work (in the first instance, and then primary prevention targeted at high-risk patients, too). The illustration in Box 4.11 below is a calculation that you might use when planning how to allocate time for nurse-led secondary prevention clinics.

Box 4.11 Nurse time for secondary prevention clinics – an illustration for a practice with 10 000 patients

If it is assumed:

- that each patient will require 30 minutes of time each year (either one 30-minute or two 15-minute slots) and
- there are 438 patients with angina or previous myocardial infarction in a practice with 10 000 patients

then: $\dfrac{438 \times 30}{60} = 219$ hours per year $= 4.2$ hours per week.

The following points should be noted.

1 If practices run clinics with 30-minute consultation slots and 30 minutes for follow-up, then this means 8.4 hours a week.
2 Practices with high rates of coronary heart disease or an older practice population will have greater numbers of patients, the reverse being true for lower coronary heart disease rates and younger populations.
3 In reality, because of the difficulty of establishing 100% complete registers and not all people attending clinics, the actual numbers followed up will be fewer.
4 Practices will also require additional administration time (letters, audit, etc.), e.g. 15–30 minutes per patient.

Advantages and disadvantages of nurse-led secondary prevention CHD clinics

Advantages

- More time is available for a comprehensive assessment of patients' needs.
- Nurses are generally better than doctors at delivering protocol-based care.
- These clinics allow for a proactive approach, and patients have time to prepare for the consultation.
- There is no distraction from unrelated patient problems.
- There is the potential to reduce GP workload, as patients may consult GPs less about non-medical aspects (e.g. general lifestyle issues) of CHD management in routine consultations, and from the prevention of future complications.
- There is better co-ordination of patient care between the primary and secondary care sectors. A patient may have to attend hospital out-patients and their general practitioner for the same issues, whereas the nurse clinic may reduce this duplication.
- There is evidence to indicate that nurse clinic-based care for CHD secondary prevention is more effective in modifying risk than 'normal' care.

Disadvantages

- It may be necessary to secure resources for additional nurse time.
- There may be duplication between aspects of the nurse clinic consultations and routine consultations with the GP.
- The workloads of GPs and the practice team may be increased because unmet patient needs may be identified.
- It may be difficult to organise clinics in smaller practices because of insufficient numbers of patients.
- Patients might find it difficult to attend specific clinic times.
- Focusing on CHD may encourage a less holistic approach to patient care.

Setting up a nurse-led secondary prevention CHD clinic

1 Establish a CHD register (see previous section).
2 Discuss within the primary care team the pros and cons of setting

up a nurse-led clinic, and consider other options such as opportunistic screening by a GP or a GP clinic. Seek examples of good practice locally from the PCO or local CHD lead.

3   Identify the numbers of patients on the CHD register. For secondary prevention, only patients with angina and those who have had a previous myocardial infarction should be included. This will limit numbers and target those at highest risk. Compare your numbers with the prevalence data given for a typical practice population of 10 000 people in Appendix 2.

4   Agree a template/protocol to be used in the clinic. Collate evidence-based advice and resource materials for patients.

5   Discuss the role of the nurse in relation to prescribing and how medical advice can be sought either during the clinic or at follow-up afterwards.

6   Consider options for the length/venue and frequency of the clinic.

7   Patients could be invited to attend in specific clinic slots or asked to make an appointment to see the nurse when convenient. Consider the factors that affect uptake, such as the ability of patients to attend (e.g. many working men may find it difficult to attend in the morning).

8   Agree an approach for collating audit data. The NSF identifies a minimum information set for audit that was summarised in Box 4.8 (see the NSF document itself for full details[2]).

9   Set evaluation parameters. For example, measure how well the clinics are running from a practical perspective (convenience to patients, and the proportion of patients invited who attend).

10 Pilot your service and review how you are doing.

A detailed example of a protocol for a nurse-led clinic for the secondary prevention of coronary heart disease

This protocol has been modified and then reproduced with the permission of North Stoke Primary Care Trust.

The following working example, on pages 61 to 65, has been developed by a primary care trust in the West Midlands. It describes the clinic protocol and the proposed audit parameters.

Aims

This protocol aims to achieve the NSF target:

> *To identify all patients with established cardiovascular disease and offer them comprehensive advice and appropriate treatment to reduce their risks.*

Stage 1 – identification

The first priority is to deal with patients with established arterial disease.

A register of all patients with cardiovascular disease will be maintained for the following:

- ischaemic heart disease
- myocardial infarction
- angina
- coronary artery bypass graft or angioplasty
- arteriosclerosis and peripheral vascular disease.

A separate register will include patients with cerebrovascular disease, stroke and transient cerebral ischaemia. The computer also maintains a register of patients with hypertension.

These registers will be maintained by:

- summarising all records, including new records entering the practice
- entering diagnoses from hospital discharge and out-patient reports
- entries made at the time of diagnosis in surgery.

(*See* Appendix 1 for a full list of Read codes.)

Stage 2 – assessment

All patients with arterial disease should have a full assessment.

Blood pressure should be measured in the sitting position, after the patient has been resting for 5 minutes, using an appropriate cuff size. Diastolic pressure should be phase 5, and blood pressure should be read to the nearest 2 mmHg. *It should be taken twice at each visit.*

Blood tests for urea and electrolytes, full blood count, total and HDL cholesterol, glucose and liver function tests should be performed annually.

Urinalysis should be performed by dipstick testing annually.

Transfer any newly diagnosed hypertensives on to the hypertension protocol.

With regard to blood lipids, total and HDL cholesterol will be measured fasting ideally, or non-fasting followed by fasting if raised.

If the total cholesterol concentration is <5 mmol/L, reassure the patient. If total cholesterol is > 5 mmol/L, refer them back to the doctor for treatment.

Stage 3 – assessment of risk

All patients with evidence of arterial disease, including previous myocardial infarct, angina, peripheral artery disease or cerebrovascular disease, are at high risk of subsequent events and should receive advice and treatment to reduce that risk.

Use the standard ischaemic heart disease template on your practice computer.

Stage 4 – lifestyle advice

All patients will be offered lifestyle advice as appropriate. Patients will be advised to reduce their cardiovascular risk by:

- stopping smoking
- eating a prudent diet, following the Committee on Medical Aspects of Food Policy (COMA) recommendations (i.e. low in saturated fat, supplemented with polyunsaturated fats and fish oils, and high in fresh fruit and vegetables)
- being moderately physically active
- keeping alcohol consumption below the recommended limits of up to 3–4 units per day for men and up to 2–3 units per day for women.

The lifestyle advice will follow a patient-centred approach with four stages:

1 eliciting the patients' views, beliefs and readiness to change
2 explaining the nature of and reasons for advice
3 negotiating and agreeing goals
4 supporting the patient in achieving and maintaining change, and reinforcing this with appropriate health promotion materials.

Stage 5 – management of risk factors

- *Smokers*: patients who actively wish to stop smoking should be offered detailed advice, including nicotine replacement therapy (or bupropion if appropriate) and follow-up.
- *Aspirin*: all patients with arterial disease should be advised to take 75 mg aspirin daily unless this is contraindicated. If it is contraindicated, refer them to the GP for advice.
- *Lifestyle advice*: all patients with CHD should receive appropriate lifestyle advice, with particular emphasis on weight reduction,

moderate alcohol intake and physical activity to reduce blood pressure, and smoking cessation and appropriate diet to reduce CHD risk.
- *Follow-up*: this should take place monthly until controlled or maximal therapy is established, and then six-monthly. All patients should have a full reassessment every five years. Patients on diuretics or ACE inhibitors should have their urine and electrolytes measured annually.

Indications for referral to GP

These include the following:

- new symptoms (e.g. chest pain, increasing shortness of breath, claudication). Urgency will depend on the nature of the symptoms
- poor control of blood pressure or lipids. Check adherence to treatment and either repeat the measurements or refer the patient back, depending on the levels
- side-effects, anxieties or difficulty in adhering to medication. Arrange a routine appointment as appropriate.

Audit requirements. Protocol audit – NSF

The performance of the programme will be reviewed annually. This review will include the following:

1   completeness of the arterial disease, cerebrovascular disease and hypertension registers by comparison with published prevalence and by cross-checks with diagnostic codes and prescribing. This should include the number identified, and comparison of percentage figures with others' prevalence data (*see* Appendix 2 for age–gender distribution of coronary vascular diseases in a typical practice of 10 000 patients)
2   recording of risk factors and levels of control in patients on the registers, including smoking habit, blood pressure, body mass index, physical activity and cholesterol, as well as general recording of Read codes and consistency, etc.
3   clinic attendance, and the number of patients on the register who have not been seen for > 12 months
4   prescribing rates for aspirin and lipid-lowering drugs for patients on the registers

5   screening – the proportions of the population, divided by sex and 10-year age groups, with recordings of:
    • blood pressure
    • smoking habit
    • significant family history.

Roles and responsibilities of the primary care organisation and primary healthcare team members

These suggestions are intended to serve as ideas for you, and are not necessarily comprehensive.

Primary care organisations

Primary care organisations need to ensure that the appropriate infrastructure is in place to achieve the NSF standards and milestones.

The PCO should provide leadership, undertake an assessment of baseline needs within the practices, support change and evaluate progress.

Leadership

To gain a critical mass of commitment within the PCO, you might:

• identify champions within the PCO and primary care teams
• establish local PCO workshops to communicate key messages
• assess barriers and opportunities for change
• provide a link with local general practice health promotion schemes
• provide incentives such as resources for practices (e.g. securing funding from pharmaceutical companies, meeting training needs and offering other support, etc.).

Assessing the baseline

This could be achieved either through a series of individual practice visits by representatives of the PCO, or by means of a postal survey or telephone interviews, etc.

A tool to assess baseline: The baseline assessment described in Box 4.12 is one that any primary care organisation or individual general practice might use to gain an overview of how well organised the systems and procedures are for chronic disease management, including CHD.

The methods used to assess the baseline could include the following:

- practice visits by a member of the PCO, either specifically for this purpose or as part of routine visits by the PCO to the practice
- telephone or postal questionnaires
- a combination of approaches to supplement the existing data that the PCO possesses about practice performance.

Box 4.12 Example of a baseline assessment that a primary care organisation or individual practice might use to assess their state of readiness for providing systematically high-quality coronary heart disease care and services (reproduced by kind permission of East Staffordshire Primary Care Group)

PCOs should complete as much information as possible before forwarding the assessment to individual practices, to avoid unnecessary duplication of data collection.

If you do not have any accurate information and wish to make a 'guesstimate', please indicate this.

1   What is your total practice population? _____
2   What percentage of your practice population is:
      (a) Urban?   ___%
      (b) Rural?   ___%
      (c) Over 65 years?   ___%
      (d) Social classes 4 or 5?   ___%
      (e) Minority groups?   ___%
3   Do you have a computer-based clinical system?   Y/N
        If Yes, which system do you use?   _____
4   Do you have an established disease register for:
      (a) CHD?   Y/N   Prevalence   ___%
      (b) At risk?   Y/N   Prevalence   ___%
      (c) PVD?   Y/N   Prevalence   ___%
      (d) CVA?   Y/N   Prevalence   ___%
      (e) HF?   Y/N   Prevalence   ___%
      (f) Other?   Y/N   Prevalence   ___%
      Type of register/s _____
5   How do you maintain your register?
      (a) Add new patients opportunistically   Y/N
      (b) Add patients newly diagnosed from hospital   Y/N

     (c) Remove patients who have died   Y/N
     (d) Remove patients who have moved away   Y/N
     (e) Do you use the clinical system for this purpose? Y/N

6   Who is responsible for the maintenance of the register in the practice?
     (a) Practice manager   Y/N
     (b) Practice nurse   Y/N
     (c) GP   Y/N
     (d) Other   Y/N
     (e) Named person is: _____

7   Do you use the Framingham risk calculation for assessing patients at risk of developing CHD?   Y/N

8   Is this a computer-based tool?   Y/N

9   Do you use a Read-coded template for CHD?   Y/N
     Which one do you use? _____
     (a) PCO template   Y/N
     (b) Extended template based on NSF for CHD   Y/N

10 Who is the lead for CHD in your practice? _____

11 Do you have a protocol of care for patients with:
     (a) CHD?   Y/N
     (b) PVD?   Y/N
     (c) CVA?   Y/N
     (d) HF?   Y/N

12 Have you summarised patient notes?   Y/N
     If Yes, what percentage is summarised? ___%

13 What proportion of these summarised notes of the total population are:
     (a) Computerised?   ___%
     (b) Paper based (Lloyd George/A4)?   __/__%
     (c) Both?   ___%

14 Do you have records of patients who are on long-term drug therapies?   Y/N
     (a) What percentage of total population of the above are computerised?   ___%
     (b) What percentage of total population of the above are on paper   ___%

15 In what percentage of the practice notes are all medical records and correspondence in date order?   ___%
     How has this been achieved and by whom?

16 Do you run coronary heart disease clinics?   Y/N
17 How are these run?
         (a) Nurse led   Y/N
         (b) Doctor led   Y/N
         (c) Simultaneous GP and practice nurse   Y/N
18 Practices in this primary care organisation have a general agreement to share clinical data. Please confirm that you will provide audit data collected within the practice for collation by PCO: Y/N

Comment

Chris Oliver, clinical development facilitator for coronary heart disease for the Queens Hospital Burton and East Staffordshire PCG locality   October 2000

Providing practical support to practices

Identification of patients with coronary heart disease:

- agree definitions, including standard Read codes across the PCO (*see* examples in Appendix 1)
- assist practices through a variety of methodologies to search for patients with coronary heart disease (e.g. using drugs, using Read code, practitioner personal knowledge, hospital lists of patients admitted with a myocardial infarction)
- support practices in validating the notes to ensure that the correct patients are identified – this will probably need to be undertaken by a clinician.

Development of a template:

- develop a PCO-wide consensus and the template to be used
- ensure that the template is incorporated into various IT systems

- support practices in integrating the template into practice software
- provide technical IT support when problems arise via trouble-shooting function
- provide technical IT support when practices change computer systems.

Entering data on to computers:

- provide options for resourcing data entry
- support practices in validating data entry
- ensure that practices have arrangements for entering new patients
- ensure that practices have systems to maintain disease registers. Are primary care team members committed to this as a long-term project?

Evaluating progress

The National Service Framework requires practices to undertake quarterly audits. The NSF has also identified a set of audit data which practices need to collate. The PCO needs to support practices in extracting this data and provide PCO-wide analysis of audit data from practice computers or from paper-based registers. The PCO could also support practices in undertaking data analysis themselves, or commission it from local audit groups or others.

Other roles of the PCO include the following:

- feedback on practice performance compared to peers
- administering the GP health promotion scheme
- undertaking an assessment of resource implications (e.g. prescribing, practitioner time, etc.)
- developing a PCO action plan and supporting practices in developing their own plans
- seeking resources and support from the health authority, and training from the local university, etc.
- providing resources, materials, etc.
- offering training to GPs and nurses who will be leading the process
- providing links with exercise prescription schemes
- encouraging protocols for referral to secondary care for further investigation and management
- creating opportunities for practices to develop a common approach, particularly between smaller practices. For example, three practices working in a single health centre might agree to provide a single secondary prevention clinic
- instituting performance management and supplying progress reports.

GPs

- Provide medical input into the secondary prevention clinics within the practice as required.
- Construct and agree protocols for nurse-led secondary prevention clinics, referrals to hospital for cardiac assessment, etc.
- Undertake assessment of patients' needs and follow-up management through opportunistic consultations in the practice as an alternative to a nurse-led secondary prevention clinic.

Primary care nurses

- Run nurse-led secondary prevention clinics for coronary heart disease.
- Work to protocols for the management of CHD secondary prevention.
- Contribute to maintaining disease registers.
- Be able to give patients with established heart disease accurate advice about their risks, and information about best practice.

Practice managers

- Ensure that there is a practice plan for implementing Standard 3 and the other Standards.
- Ensure that there is an IT infrastructure for the development of disease registers.
- Ensure that the training needs of staff for computer skills and clinical expertise are identified and met.

Receptionists

- Ensure that the CHD secondary prevention approach within the practice is widely publicised to patients.
- Lead on updating disease registers.
- Adhere to the practice protocol for providing repeat medication and review.

Tips for secondary prevention

1   Do not establish paper-based registers to meet a short-term target. Think of long- term solutions and develop appropriate IT systems for registers.

2   Do not develop your own protocols, templates, Read code definitions, audit tools, etc. Borrow, copy or adapt others.

3   Before establishing nurse-led clinics, make a case for resources for additional nursing time.

4   Invest in nurse training (e.g. British Heart Save Course) (*see* Appendix 4 for details).

5   In order to identify all patients with coronary heart disease, use a variety of strategies, including posters in the surgery and possibly articles in local newspapers, to promote self-identification.

6   Many of those attending diabetic clinics will have coronary heart disease or be at high-risk of CHD. Use the CHD template in diabetic clinics where appropriate.

7   Consider running nurse-led coronary heart disease clinics in parallel with a normal routine GP surgery. A patient could have a 20-minute appointment with a nurse, followed by 10-minute appointment with the GP in a parallel surgery.

8   Ask patients to come in a week before their appointment with the nurse-led coronary heart disease clinic for a prescribed set of blood tests. Their results will then be available for the comprehensive assessment in the nurse-led clinic.

9   Nurses running the coronary heart disease clinics will need peer support, which may be available either from local nurses or from the local specialist nurses in hospital cardiac rehabilitation units.

10 Use an evidence-based approach for providing lifestyle advice. A set of British Heart Foundation booklets is available as a series on lifestyle issues (exercise, diet, smoking, hyperlipidaemia, etc.).

11 Empower patients to take responsibility for managing their condition through patient-held treatment plans (see the CHD NSF[2] for an example).

12 Patients may well be asked to adhere to a multitude of drugs with complex regimes. Agree and monitor adherence through a realistic plan which suits the individual patient. It is worth remembering that patients with cancer are usually willing to comply with complex and unpleasant therapeutic regimes, and that many patients with CHD are at similar risk of death and morbidity.

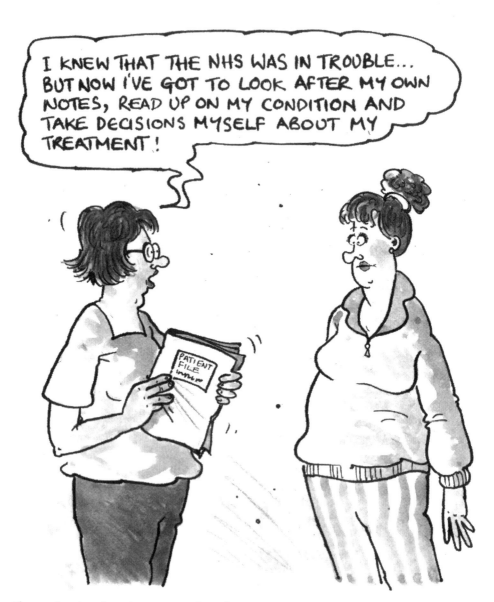

If you don't take time to explain best practice, it may be misconstrued.

CHAPTER 5

Primary prevention targeted at high-risk groups in primary care

People with hypertension, high cholesterol levels or diabetes are at much higher risk of developing coronary heart disease than the general population.

Box 5.1 Standard 4 of the NSF

General practitioners and primary healthcare teams should identify all people at significant risk of cardiovascular disease but who have not yet developed symptoms, and offer them appropriate advice and treatment to reduce their risks.

Primary prevention can be focused on a smaller group of people who are at high risk of developing coronary heart disease. Efforts should be made to modify individuals' high risk through personalised approaches. For instance, a personal approach for people with diabetes mellitus would include targeting other coexisting multiple predisposing factors (e.g. smoking, hypertension and high cholesterol levels) that put them at a higher risk of a cardiac event occurring in the future than some other patients with existing coronary heart disease.

Box 5.2 Estimated numbers of high-risk patients in a typical practice with 10 000 patients[53]

Estimated proportion of the population	Estimated numbers of patients
A 10-year 30% or higher risk of a coronary event would identify 3.4% of the population aged 35–69 for preventative treatment	142
Lowering the prevention threshold to 15% or more for a risk of a coronary event occurring in the next 10 years would identify 25% of the population	1095
If all patients at such a 15% or higher CHD risk were to be identified using the Sheffield Table,[54] then an estimated 70% of the population aged 35–64 years would need to be screened.	2619 require screening

---

Appendix 2 lists more data, giving a gender–age breakdown of patients with various conditions related to coronary heart disease, in a typical patient population of 10 000.

Box 5.3 Nurse led clinic for primary, secondary and tertiary prevention of heart disease and the use of IT decision support[27]

One practice uses a comprehensive computerised system for the opportunistic and systematic management of smoking, blood pressure, hypertension, cholesterol and chronic heart failure. The practice has developed a set of evidence-based standards to prevent and effectively manage heart disease. Information for clinical governance and audit is also collected with no additional effort on the part of the clinician.

Contact: Bewdley Medical Centre. Tel: 01299 402157.

Patients who are at high risk of developing coronary heart disease should receive the following:[2]

1 an assessment and quantification of their risk status

2   an explanation of their risk status and its implications
3   an evidence-based programme of both therapeutic and non-therapeutic interventions aiming to reduce risk
4   appropriate review and follow-up arrangements
5   a reduction in their individual risk of developing heart disease.

Risk factors

Age

Elderly people have the same risk factors for coronary heart disease as the general population, although the association between risk factors and CHD may be less strong. The risk of developing coronary heart disease increases with age. As CHD is much more common in the elderly, they are as likely to benefit from preventative measures as younger people, if not more so.

We need evidence from research trials to make fair decisions about treating older people with primary prevention therapy. Otherwise, value judgements will come into play when balancing priorities for treating individuals on the basis of age and risk status alone.

Controlling hypertension is probably the most important modifiable risk factor for CHD in elderly people.

Gender

Very few trials have examined the risk factor status, intervention and outcomes in women. Many of the risk assessment tools extrapolate the results from trials including men to women.

Data from the General Practice Research Database show that although overall treatment rates have improved in both men and women with CHD, women are still not prescribed drugs as often as men.[55]

Important gender differences and similarities include the following:

* higher rates of obesity, higher total cholesterol, and more frequently occurring diabetes in women aged over 55 years
* more frequent hypertension in women aged over 65 years than in men of similar age
* the onset of CHD in women lags about 10 years behind that in men

- women under 65 years of age have one-third of the CHD mortality rate for men of a similar age
- women more commonly present with angina, and men more commonly present with myocardial infarction
- women are as likely as men to reinfarct after a myocardial infarction. Some studies have suggested that there is a poorer prognosis for women post-myocardial infarction. This may be because some hospitals tend to admit fewer female patients to the coronary care unit,[15] and women tend to present at an older age
- women are at least as likely to benefit from lipid-lowering drug therapy as men.

Minority ethnic groups

People from South Asia living in the UK have a much higher (40% higher) risk of developing heart disease than white people in the UK, whilst for people of African-Caribbean origin the risk is up to 50% lower, but the risk of hypertension is higher.

Diabetes

Diabetes increases the risk of developing heart disease up to fivefold, and heart disease is one of the most important causes of death among people with diabetes.[40] Individuals with diabetes are also more likely to suffer from hypertension, hyperlipidaemia, heart failure and cardiogenic shock.

Good control of blood sugar will reduce the microvascular complications of diabetes, and it is critical to modify risk factors, particularly smoking, hyperlipidaemia and high blood pressure.[48]

There is a high absolute risk for cardiovascular disease in patients with diabetes, which suggests that there is a greater benefit from lipid-lowering therapy in people with diabetes compared with those without diabetes for a given cholesterol/HDL ratio.[56] There is some evidence to suggest that the available risk assessment methods may underestimate diabetic CHD with type 1 individuals. It seems as if the HDL in type 1 diabetes does not confer the same degree of protection against CHD as it does for people without diabetes. Therefore lipid-lowering therapy should be considered at a lower risk threshold in these individuals.[49]

Familial hypercholesterolaemia

Familial hypercholesterolaemia is an autosomal-dominant condition that affects about one in 500 of the UK population. These individuals need to be treated aggressively with dietary advice and lipid-lowering therapy. Referral to a specialist clinic is recommended.

Risk assessment

Much of the available information on risk is derived from the Framingham study, which examined 5000 people living in an American suburb and followed them up for 30 years. The study includes data on a range of coronary heart disease risk factors, such as blood pressure, smoking and lipid concentration, together with causes of death and disease, and the findings are used to predict death or major vascular events.

In the UK as well as in the USA the standard adopted for expressing risk is 'the risk of a coronary heart disease event in 10 years (either myocardial infarction death or non-fatal myocardial infarction)'.

The risk data from the Framingham study are similar to those from other studies that have been conducted in Northern Europe, but somewhat overestimate the risk compared with the British Regional Heart study.[57]

Prediction of risk using the multiple risk factors from these studies is much better than that using single factors alone to determine prognoses. In practice it has been found that the equation predicting coronary heart disease events based on the Framingham data is also a reasonable predictor of stroke and an accurate predictor of coronary heart disease plus stroke.[53]

Tools to assist the measurement of risk

There are a range of charts and tables based on the Framingham data, as well as numerous software packages which calculate risk in the clinical setting. Risk charts[54] include:

- the Sheffield Table
- the New Zealand Guidelines
- the Joint British Chart.

A recent study comparing the Sheffield Table and the Joint British Chart scoring method found that:

- nurses interpreted the New Zealand Guidelines and the Joint British Chart more accurately than the Sheffield Table
- doctors and nurses prefer the New Zealand Guidelines and the Joint British Chart to the Sheffield Table.

Any software needs to be easy to use and provide clinicians with rapid information at the point of decision making. One example is the Egton Medical Information Systems (EMIS) clinical computer system, which uses the Framingham equations with a clinical system, thus avoiding the need to enter data twice.

There are also a range of computer-based risk assessment packages which are available on the Internet or can be used as floppy disks, such as http://cebm.jr2.ox.ac.uk/docs/prognosis.html

Problems with risk predictors include the following.

- Risk predictions can be flawed when some of the variables are at their extremes.
- Family history is not considered in the equations, and therefore risks are likely to be greater than predicted.
- Underestimation of the risk of those with heterozygous familial high blood cholesterol hypercholesterolaemia may occur.
- Underestimation of the risk for South Asians living in the UK and those on low incomes may occur.

Risk assessment tools should be an adjunct to clinical judgement, so that individual circumstances are considered when making clinical management decisions.

The effectiveness of primary prevention interventions for those at high risk of developing coronary heart disease

Lifestyle risk factors

Concentrate on lifestyle interventions as a priority, particularly in those patients whose absolute coronary heart disease risk is not sufficient to warrant drug therapy.

Smoking cessation support is critical, and the risk of developing coronary heart disease is halved after one year in smokers who quit. However, it may take 10 years of not smoking to reach the reduced risk level of those individuals who have never smoked.

Physical activity is strongly associated with a lower risk of coronary heart disease. The largest reductions in risk are in people who were previously sedentary or moderately active, compared with modest risk reductions in those people who were already vigorously active. Brisk walking or heavy gardening are particularly effective, especially if sustained for long periods.

Diet plays an important role, with the amount of saturated fat being the most important determinant. Oily fish and monounsaturated fatty acids are protective against coronary heart disease, and increased consumption of fruit and vegetables may also be protective.

Current evidence suggests that foods (e.g. margarines) enriched with stanol esters or plant sterols also reduce cholesterol concentrations in those who consume an average-cholesterol diet, but are not as effective in those on a low-fat diet.

Reductions in dietary salt lead to reduced hypertension and thus reduced CHD risk, too. A body mass index (BMI) of less than 25 is the goal.

Light to moderate drinkers have lower CHD mortality than heavy drinkers.

For more details about recommended lifestyles, *see* Chapter 2.

Therapeutic interventions

Lipid-lowering drugs

There have been two randomised controlled primary prevention trials involving pravastatin and lovastatin.[13,14,15,58] Both of these trials showed significant reductions in cardiac event rates of around a third. One showed a reduction in all-cause mortality, but this was of borderline statistical significance.

There have been no long-term controlled trials involving atorva-statin, cerivastatin or fluvastatin.

Two trials involving fibrates have showed reductions in CHD events. Fibrates are not recommended as first-line lipid-lowering interventions because of concerns about adverse effects.[15]

Aspirin

The Scottish SIGN guidelines recommend that aspirin is taken by all patients whose risk is high enough to justify the use of lipid-lowering drugs.[15]

At the 15% risk threshold – that is, the risk of a CHD event occurring in the next 10 years – aspirin does reduce the risk of coronary events, but 60 people would need to be treated for five years to avoid one coronary or stroke event. This has to be balanced against the risk of gastrointestinal haemorrhage. Therefore it is recommended that aspirin should be limited to those people who are at or above the 30% risk threshold.

Hypertension and high-risk patients

The updated British Hypertension Society guidelines recognise the importance of cardiac risk, particularly for mild hypertension.[59] The guidelines recommend the use of the Cardiac Risk Assessor computer program developed by the Joint British Societies.

Current guidelines for deciding whether and how to treat people with raised blood pressure are summarised in Boxes 5.4 and 5.5, and Figure 5.1.

Box 5.4 Thresholds and treatment targets for antihypertensive drug therapy

- Drug therapy should be started in all patients with sustained systolic blood pressures of >160 mmHg or sustained diastolic blood pressures of >100 mmHg, despite non-pharmacological measures.
- Drug treatment is also indicated in patients with sustained systolic blood pressure of 140–159 mmHg or diastolic blood pressure of 90–99 mmHg if target organ damage is present, or if there is evidence of established cardiovascular disease or diabetes, or the 10-year CHD risk is $>15\%$.
- For most patients, a target of <140 mmHg systolic blood pressure and <85 mmHg diastolic blood pressure is recommended. For patients with diabetes, a lower target of $<140/80$ mmHg is recommended.

Adapted from the British Hypertension Society guidelines.[59]

The role of ACE inhibitors (ramipril) in relation to primary prevention has been amended following the HOPE study and is described in Box 4.2.[47]

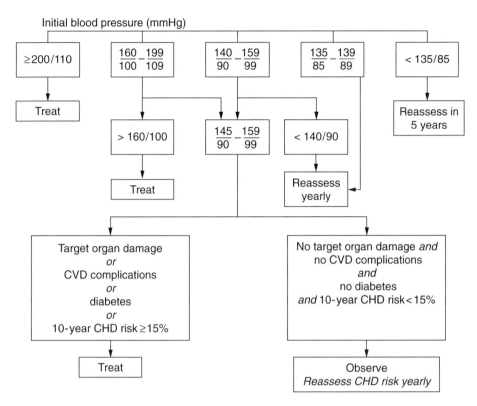

Figure 5.1: Flow diagram for antihypertensive drug therapy and cardiac risk (from Joint British Societies CHD Risk Chart[49]).

Box 5.5 Antihypertensive drug treatment[49]

- Use a low dose of thiazide as first-line treatment, unless there is a contraindication or a compelling indication for another class of drug.
- The choice of drug will depend on the relative indications and contraindications in the individual patient.
- Less than half of all people with hypertension will be controlled on monotherapy, and one-third will require three or more drugs.

Hormone replacement therapy (HRT)

The evidence for the effectiveness of HRT in the prevention of coronary heart disease is inconclusive.

What are the priorities for treatment in primary prevention?

In decreasing order of priority of effort and resources, these are as follows.

1 Promote healthy lifestyles – promote physical activity, reduce alcohol intake and support smoking cessation.
2 Prioritise people with existing coronary heart disease for lipid-lowering therapy (i.e. institute secondary prevention before primary prevention).
3 Control hypertension.
4 Institute primary preventative measures, including the prescribing of statins for everyone with a risk of 30% or higher of a CHD event occurring in the next 10 years.[54,60] The recommended age limits are described below. A practical approach might be to include everyone aged under 75 years, and to treat those aged over 75 years on a case-by-case basis.
5 Target individuals with at least a 15% risk of a CHD event occurring in the next 10 years for advice on lifestyle, check on cholesterol, control of blood pressure and other primary preventative interventions.

Treating high-risk individuals

Interventions with drugs can reduce the risk of coronary heart disease events and all-cause mortality in individuals with a risk of as low as 6% for a CHD event occurring over the next 10 years. If a programme was implemented to identify all patients with this level of risk and to offer them interventions, it would be an enormous drain on NHS resources which could not be justified at present. Therefore a staged approach is recommended in both the NSF and the Joint British Recommendations on prevention of coronary heart disease in general practice.

Box 5.6

Using the 30% 10-year risk threshold for a practice of 10 000 patients, 293 patients would require secondary prevention (all ages), and 56 patients (age 35–69 years) would be eligible for primary prevention.

Age

The Joint British Recommendations recommend that the upper age limit for initiating lipid-lowering medication should be 75 years, and that for primary prevention it should be 69 years.[49] The recommendation from the Scottish Intercollegiate Guidelines Network is that elderly patients on existing lipid-lowering therapy should not have their drugs stopped on account of age. However, until further evidence is obtained from trials, the evidence of a benefit from using lipid-lowering drugs for primary prevention of CHD in men and women who are older than 70 years remains uncertain (see point 4 in the above list of priorities).

Cost implications

The broad national cost implications for treating at a 30% risk threshold over 10 years would require 3.4% of the population aged 35–69 years to be treated for primary prevention and 4.8% for secondary prevention, giving a total of 8.2% of the population. The total cost would be around £1 billion per annum. The costs include those of prescribing, screening and primary care services.

Box 5.7

It has been estimated that the cost of statins alone (for treating at or above the 30% risk level) is £200 000 for secondary prevention and £50 000 for primary prevention in a practice of 10 000 patients.[61]

Primary care costs of primary prevention include the following:

- doctor and nurse time
- staff administrative costs for setting up a recall system
- laboratory costs for monitoring the population
- prescribing costs.

The huge costs could be mitigated by several factors.

- Targeting patients will be a gradual process.
- Not all high-risk patients may be identified in practice.
- There will be newer, more cost-effective drugs.

- There will be price reductions when generic statins become available.
- Patients' adherence to treatment will be markedly lower in the 'real world' than in research trials where volunteers are generally well motivated.

Box 5.8

If this preventative treatment threshold was lowered to 15%, then a quarter of the population should be considered for aspirin, statins or hypertensive therapy. The cost to the NHS drug budgets alone would be just under £3 billion.

How should those with at least a 30% risk of a CHD event over 10 years be identified?

The first step in achieving Standard 4 of the NSF[2] will be to identify those patients who are at high risk. One of the problems with primary prevention in high-risk individuals is that, in order to identify them, a form of screening is required either through opportunistic checks in routine consultations or as new patients register with the surgery.

Potentially the whole of the UK population could be screened for risk, as the UK has one of the highest rates of heart disease in the western world, and most heart-related deaths actually occur in people who are not in the highest-risk categories.

Box 5.9

Primary prevention through a generalised screening programme poses enormous challenges and is impractical because of the workload implications. Identifying everyone with a risk of 15% or higher would involve measuring lipid levels in 70% of the population aged 35–64 years.[53]

Treating everyone at or above the 30% risk level would mean screening 35 men and 200 women aged between 35 and 64 years in order to identify one individual who was at high risk. This is often referred to as the 'numbers needed to screen' (NNS). The NNS is much higher for women (*see* Box 5.10).

An alternative approach recommended in the Scottish SIGN Guidelines[15] for identifying patients at 30% risk is to limit screening to individuals with:

- diabetes, including those with impaired glucose tolerance
- hypertension
- a family history of premature CHD (first-degree male relatives under 55 years of age and female relatives under 65 years)
- clinical signs of hyperlipidaemia
- a history of smoking.

The NSF also recommends prioritising people with established diagnoses of diabetes and hypertension, rather than unselected screening of the whole population. The benefits of such a staged approach are that those at highest risk are targeted first, and the burden on primary care of organising and delivering care is managed in a stepwise fashion.

Using this approach, every ninth patient with hypertension and every eighth patient with diabetes will have an absolute risk higher than 3% per annum, whilst around 25 smokers would need to be screened in order to identify one person at high risk, as Box 5.10 shows.

Box 5.10 Numbers of patients needed to screen (NNS) to identify those at higher than 30% risk over 10 years[15]

Diabetes
Males	6
Females	11
Males and females	8

Hypertension
Males	5
Females	22
Males and females	9

Smoking
Males	12
Females	107
Males and females	25

Concentrating on high-risk groups leads to more manageable numbers needed to screen. However, the overall implications with regard to workload are still enormous for primary care, especially with the inclusion of smokers in the categories to be screened.

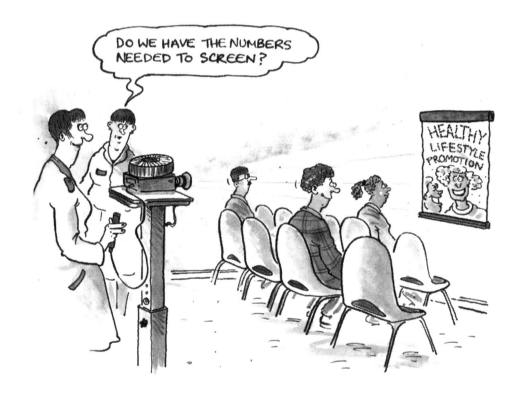

The cost-effectiveness and management implications for primary care have yet to be determined for these various approaches. A practice should anticipate the likely impact of any planned primary prevention programme before embarking on it, in terms of the following:

- the numbers of people to be screened
- the pace at which the programme is undertaken (time-scales)
- prescribing costs
- the costs of assessing risk and providing effective interventions
- training implications.

Which tests?

The best lipid predictor of coronary heart disease is the ratio of total cholesterol to HDL cholesterol.

Measure triglyceride after a 12-hour fast in order to obtain an accurate measurement of baseline levels.

Exclude secondary causes of high lipids by checking the following:

- urea, creatinine and electrolyes
- urinanalysis
- fasting glucose
- liver function tests
- thyroid-stimulating hormone.

Box 5.11 Outreach cardiology service using teleconferencing[27]

The Hampstead Group Practice has developed a virtual-outreach cardiology service jointly with a local hospital using a teleconferencing facility. Joint medical consultations occur involving the general practitioner, the consultant, the patient and practice nurses.

An outreach clinic is run by a practice nurse, and the hospital specialist attends monthly to review patients with the GP.

Contact Practice Manager: Tel: 020 7435 4000

Target cholesterol levels

The data from some of the trials suggest that there may be little to be gained in primary prevention by lowering total serum cholesterol levels much below 5.0 mmol/L.[62] Measurement of HDL/LDL ratios assumes more importance in primary prevention.

Implementation of primary prevention programmes

After targeting secondary prevention programmes at those with established heart disease, the following steps should be followed.

1 Develop a costed practice implementation plan.
2 Agree on a prevention and disease management protocol.
3 Expand the secondary prevention register to incorporate people who are at high risk.
4 Provide structured care to people at high risk of developing CHD. Target those with diabetes and hypertension first.
5 Evaluate your performance – identifying high-risk patients, controlling their risks, etc.

The check-list in Box 5.12 gives a detailed description of the issues that need to be considered when formulating the plan.

Box 5.12 Check-list of issues that need to be considered when developing a practice plan for identifying and treating patients at high risk of developing CHD

- Have all patients with coronary heart disease been identified, reviewed and managed according to evidence-based guidelines? That is, has secondary prevention been addressed first?
- How many patients without CHD have had their risk assessed and are undergoing a primary prevention treatment programme? How many patients below the 30% 10-year risk threshold are being treated?
- How will the 30% risk at 10 years be assessed? What tools will be used?
- How will primary prevention patients be identified? Will the recommendations for identifying diabetic and hypertensive patients at a higher than 30% 10-year risk be implemented first?
- How many diabetic patients and hypertensive patients will need to be screened and how many high-risk patients will be identified following such a screening programme?

- Over what time period will these patients be identified?
- Can the existing practice CHD clinic be modified to deal with primary prevention patients?
- What will be the prescribing implications, particularly for statins and ACE-inhibitor prescribing?
- What will be the impact of the additional work upon support services such as smoking cessation clinics, dietary support, exercise prescription schemes, etc.?
- Will the existing IT templates need to be modified?
- What other IT implications will there be?
- What will be the arrangements for cholesterol testing?
- What will be the additional training requirements?
- What additional protocols will be required for related issues (e.g. treatment of hypertension and atrial fibrillation)?
- What cut-off value for age will be used for primary prevention?
- Over what time-scales will this plan be implemented?
- What will be the manpower implications (additional GP, nursing and administration time)?
- What protocols will need to be agreed with others (e.g. local biochemists, endocrinologists and cardiologists)?

Agree disease management protocols[15]

Guidelines should address the following:

- screening
- lifestyle, counselling and follow-up
- therapeutic interventions
- monitoring and review.

Ideally, protocols need to be agreed between members of the primary care team, PCO representatives, local cardiologists and local biochemists/endocrinologists.

Development of a primary prevention register

Expand the disease register for secondary prevention to include those at high-risk of developing a CHD event over a 10-year period. Include those with diabetes, hypertension or of South Asian descent.

The following minimum information about risk factors should be included on the risk register:

- smoking status
- physical activity profile
- body mass index
- blood pressure
- serum cholesterol
- blood glucose or HbAlc (for those with diabetes).

Box 5.13 Development of a primary prevention disease register initially targeting patients with diabetes and hypertension

Many practices have established diabetic registers as part of chronic disease management programmes. If a diabetic register exists within the practice, then it will greatly facilitate the identification of individuals with diabetes at high risk of developing coronary heart disease. Either a manual approach, such as the use of the Sheffield Tables on paper charts, or computerised risk-assessment tools could be used to assess the level of risk.

A similar approach could be adopted for patients with hypertension if a hypertensive register already exists or a hypertension clinic operates within the practice. In the absence of this, an opportunistic approach should be taken by members of the primary care team to assess the coronary heart disease risk as patients with hypertension consult them.

As high-risk patients are identified, their details will be entered on the primary prevention register.

Ideally, the data recorded should:

- allow calculation of coronary heart disease risk
- enable practices to aggregate and analyse the data so that it can be used to support clinical audit both within the practice and across the primary care organisation.

Provision of structured care

Co-ordinate existing clinics, such as the following:

- diabetic clinic
- well-person clinic
- dietetic/nutrition clinic

- lipid-risk clinic
- hypertension clinic
- smoking cessation clinic.

Work out model individualised programmes for people with different categories and levels of risk.

Evaluation

The following data will be required for audit:[2]

1 the number and proportion of people aged 35–74 years with an identified major risk factor for cardiovascular disease, whose 10-year absolute risk of experiencing major vascular events has been assessed and documented
2 the number and percentage of those identified as being at risk whose risk has been reduced below a particular risk threshold.

Roles and responsibilities of the primary healthcare team

These suggestions are just ideas and are not intended to be comprehensive.

Primary care organisations (PCOs)

PCOs will need to ensure that practices achieve the secondary prevention described in Standard 3 before undertaking the primary prevention programmes of Standard 4. Many practices have undertaken primary prevention in an unstructured way for years, and should be encouraged to prioritise secondary prevention.

PCOs have a public health duty to ensure that populations with the greatest need are receiving high-quality services. PCOs may need to find additional investment to help practices working in areas of high deprivation to meet Standards 3 and 4. Other roles of the PCO include the following:

- providing in-depth PCO-wide assessment of the implications of implementing Standard 4
- helping practices to assess their needs and develop realistic plans

- agreeing PCO-wide protocols between primary care professionals and hospital cardiologists and endocrinologists/biochemists
- securing resources for practices to undertake this work
- agreeing a consensus on priorities (e.g. which patients should be targeted first)
- ensuring that practices have appropriate IT facilities which enable clinicians to access information on risk at the point of decision making
- supporting practices in evaluating their progress.

GPs

GPs will need to lead the practice team in prioritising primary prevention programmes after the secondary prevention programmes are well established in the practice. In particular, they will need to:

- lead the agreement of practice protocols for prevention of CHD
- lead the action plan for establishing CHD prevention programmes
- anticipate costs of prevention and negotiate with the PCO for resources
- adhere to a structured approach to prevention programmes, rather than carrying out *ad-hoc* primary prevention activities.

Primary care nurses

- Calculate patients' risks of CHD by means of charts or software programs.
- Be able to give patients accurate and up-to-date information and advice about risk reduction.
- Adhere to practice protocols for reducing CHD risk.

Practice managers

- Ensure that the IT infrastructure is in place for assessing risk and developing registers.
- Identify staff training needs and find resources and training opportunities to address these needs.
- Negotiate with the PCO to produce information about performance that will allow locality-wide monitoring to achieve Standard 4.

Pharmacists

- Contribute to the drawing up of practice protocols for primary and secondary prevention.
- Contribute to repeat prescribing, and encourage patient compliance with prescribed treatment.
- Be able to reinforce health messages about reducing CHD risks in line with the evidence and local protocols.

CHAPTER 6

Myocardial infarction, angina and revascularisation

Acute myocardial infarction

Box 6.1 Standard 5 of the NSF

People with symptoms of a possible heart attack should receive help from an individual equipped with and appropriately trained in the use of a defibrillator within eight minutes of calling for help, to maximise the benefits of resuscitation should it be necessary.

Individuals who have symptoms of a heart attack need to be assessed rapidly, and are best managed in hospital in case they need instant cardiopulmonary resuscitation and defibrillation.

Box 6.2

Revascularisation includes coronary artery bypass graft or percutaneous transluminal coronary angioplasty.

Around 70% of all coronary heart disease deaths occur outside hospital. Ventricular fibrillation leads to many preventable deaths. Lives can be saved if a patient arrests in the presence of a person with a defibrillator. Modern defibrillators are easy to use and can be used by lay people with minimal training. The siting of defibrillators in public places such as railway stations and shopping centres is being considered.

It is debatable whether individual GPs should have defibrillators to hand when they are on call. Every GP sees around two to three patients with myocardial infarction each year, and there are far fewer cases than of cardiac arrest. It is unlikely that a defibrillator will be in the right place when it is needed. In urban areas it seems sensible to rely on an efficient ambulance service to meet the eight-minute response-time target. Rural communities should consider the possibility of having a debrillator sited locally.

Primary care team members should all be able to perform cardiopulmonary resuscitation, and they should encourage members of the public to be trained in this procedure, too.

Box 6.3 Standard 6 of the NSF

People who are thought to be suffering from a heart attack should be assessed professionally and, if indicated, should receive aspirin. Thrombolysis should be given within 60 minutes of calling for professional help.

Although there is a national trend towards the increasing use of 999 calls for chest pain, there is still considerable public misunderstanding about the urgency of obtaining expert help for prolonged chest pain.

It is extremely difficult for health professionals or the general public to make an accurate diagnosis when chest pain presents. Not all prolonged chest pain is due to ischaemia, and not all angina attacks lead to infarction.

Box 6.4 Not all protracted chest pain is a myocardial infarction[63]

One study of patients at an Accident and Emergency department illustrates the wide spectrum of types of chest pain that present. Half of the patients who presented with 'chest pain', 'angina' or 'heart attack' were admitted. Of these, one-fifth had an acute myocardial infarction, one-third had angina and the rest had a non-cardiac cause accounting for their pain.

Pre-hospital thrombolysis with anistreplase or urokinase is being piloted but is not generally available. This may have more of a place in rural areas, where there will be a delay in getting the patient to hospital.

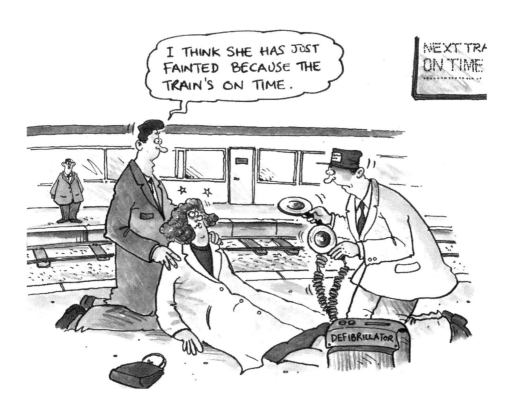

Roles and responsibilities of the primary healthcare team in acute myocardial infarction

These suggestions are just ideas and are not intended to be comprehensive.

GPs

Telephone triage – if there is the least suspicion of a heart attack, then the emergency (eight-minute response) ambulance service should be summoned. The GP should visit the patient as well in order to:

- help establish the diagnosis
- reassure the relatives
- administer analgesic drugs – intravenous diamorphine and an anti-emetic to relieve pain and distress. In the absence of a GP, most ambulance services are authorised to use nalbuphine
- ensure that an aspirin tablet is given to the patient and chewed before swallowing.

Receptionists

- The general principle is *better safe than sorry*. Receptionists must immediately refer all calls about 'chest pain', 'collapse' or 'difficulty in breathing' to the GP covering emergencies.
- Even if there is a small risk of a myocardial infarction, the ambulance should be called with a clear message that patients should be targeted for an eight-minute response. An 'urgent request' is of lower priority than the eight-minute response request; 999 calls are all treated as emergencies.

Patients

- Media campaigns and wider publicity encourage people who suspect that they or another person with chest pain are having a heart attack to seek medical help as soon as possible, by tele-phoning 999. Contacting *NHS Direct* will trigger an emergency response.

Post-myocardial infarction care[13,64,65]

Box 6.5 Standard 7 of the NSF

NHS trusts should put in place agreed protocols/systems of care so that people who are admitted to hospital with proven heart attack are appropriately assessed and offered treatments of proven clinical and cost-effectiveness to reduce their risk of disability and death.

Primary care organisations should agree the protocol for secondary prevention with local GPs, nurses and cardiologists, for those who have sustained a myocardial infarction, to ensure that the standard is being met. This is important in order to:

- ensure that drug treatment (e.g. choice of statins) is consistent
- ensure that information systems and definitions used for certain conditions are consistent with those being used within primary care, so that appropriate comparisons can be made
- give patients consistent messages across primary and secondary care settings.

Cardiac rehabilitation

Cardiac rehabilitation can reduce the death rate by 20–25% (*see* Chapter 8).

All patients should be offered a programme of cardiac rehabilitation. The programme should start in hospital and be provided by specialist multidisciplinary staff.

Medication unless contraindicated

- *Beta-blocker drugs*: protect high- and low-risk post-myocardial infarction patients against sudden death. Treatment with beta-blocker drugs after an acute myocardial infarction does not increase survival in the short term, but does have long-term benefits, which are of the order of prevention of 12 deaths for every 1000 patients treated in the first year. Therefore all patients with acute myocardial infarction should be continued indefinitely on an oral beta-blocker drug unless it is contraindicated (e.g. for people who have asthma).

- *ACE inhibitor drugs*: starting ACE inhibitors promptly after myocardial infarction reduces the death rate in both the short term and longer term – an effect that persists even if ACE inhibitors are discontinued after a few weeks.

  All patients should take an ACE inhibitor indefinitely if there are no contraindications. The evidence is most robust for taking ACE inhibitors for about six weeks after myocardial infarction, and for people who have left ventricular dysfunction.

Box 6.6

Both an ACE inhibitor and a beta-blocker should be continued indefinitely after a myocardial infarction unless there are contra-indications.

- *Aspirin*: this should be taken indefinitely if myocardial infarction or other atherosclerotic disease is confirmed. Consider clopidogrel if aspirin is contraindicated.
- *Statins*: if the patient has a cholesterol level of 5.0 mmol/L or higher, a statin should be started before discharge from hospital.
- *Warfarin*: this should be used for post-myocardial infarction (MI) patients who have permanent atrial fibrillation. People with large anterior myocardial infarcts and left ventricular aneurysms should receive warfarin for at least three months.
- *Thrombolysis*: those who survive an acute MI should be given thrombolysis, provided that the ECG meets specified criteria indicating that an MI has occurred.

Investigations

High-risk patients should be considered for coronary angiography as a preliminary to revascularisation. This patient group includes those who after myocardial infarction have angina or significant changes in an exercise ECG or isotope perfusion imaging.

Post-MI patients who also have diabetes

These patients need to have their blood pressure and blood sugar levels meticulously controlled.

Auditing Standard 7 of the NSF

By April 2002, 80–90% of patients discharged from hospital should be prescribed effective medication, especially aspirin, beta-blockers, ACE inhibitors and statins.

You should use audit to confirm that systems are in place and working, and that appropriate interventions are being offered.

Angina and revascularisation

Box 6.7 Standard 8 of the NSF

People with symptoms of angina or suspected angina should receive appropriate investigations and treatment to relieve their pain and reduce their risk of coronary events.

Box 6.8 Standard 9 of the NSF

People with angina that is increasing in frequency or severity should be referred to a cardiologist urgently or, for those at greatest risk, as an emergency.

Box 6.9 Standard 10 of the NSF

NHS trusts should put in place hospital-wide systems of care, so that patients with suspected or confirmed coronary artery disease receive timely and appropriate investigation and treatment to relieve their symptoms and reduce their risk of subsequent coronary events.

Stable angina is due to a gradual occlusion of coronary arteries by atheroma. Angina is the commonest symptom of coronary heart disease. The prevalence of stable angina is 2.6% for people over 30 years of age.

Around 22 000 new cases of angina present annually in the UK.

Deprivation has an important influence, and there is a much higher rate in deprived areas. The incidence of angina is also much higher in men. The actual incidence depends on the catchment population, as it varies widely across the UK.

Death and myocardial infarction will occur in up to 14% of individuals who present with stable angina. Those with the highest risk have three-vessel coronary disease, proximal two-vessel disease with left ventricular impairment, or left main-stem disease.

The British Cardiac Society has suggested referral to a cardiologist (or a physician with a special interest in cardiology) in the following situations:[66]

- newly diagnosed angina in patients under 70 years of age
- severe stable angina or rapidly progressing symptoms
- secondary angina from a remediable condition (e.g. anaemia or thyrotoxicosis)
- where the diagnosis is unclear (e.g. atypical history)
- unacceptable symptoms despite adequate medical therapy
- where a positive diagnosis has vocational implications (e.g. public service vehicle licence holders or pilots).

Age

There is no age limit for revascularisation procedures in the NSF. In comparison with medical treatment, there is no advantage in terms of mortality with coronary angioplasty. PTCA reduces symptoms and improves the quality of life. Coronary artery bypass surgery only improves the prognosis in selected patients. The benefits are less clear-cut in those with a high operative risk (e.g. patients who have stroke, respiratory or renal comorbidity).

The North of England evidence-based guidelines for angina[54] cover the following:

- investigation
- management of risk factors
- blood pressure management
- therapeutic interventions
- referral issues.

The guidelines recommend that all patients should have the following investigations:

- serum lipids
- haemoglobin
- thyroid function

- blood glucose
- a resting and exercise ECG.

Following this, the guidelines recommend that any risk factors should be dealt with by:

- treatment to lower cholesterol and blood pressure
- aspirin as appropriate
- a weight management programme
- dietary management
- advice to take more exercise
- smoking cessation support.

Special considerations

Most tests such as exercise ECGs are less accurate in women than in men, and the reason for this is not clearly understood. People with diabetes have an up to fivefold increased risk of dying from heart disease, and therefore those with angina need meticulous attention to their diabetes control and other risk factors. People of South Asian descent have a risk factor which is 40% higher than that for the Caucasian population in the UK, whilst individuals of African-Caribbean descent have a 25–50% lower risk than Caucasians.

Rapid-access chest pain clinics for recent-onset angina

The UK has one of the lowest coronary revascularisation rates in Europe, and often there is a long waiting list for investigations and treatment. One of the milestones within the NSF is to introduce rapid-access chest pain clinics. A total of 50 such clinics should have been established by April 2001 in England, with a national roll out after April 2002.

What this means for patients with angina

- Referral to specialist chest pain clinics and a guarantee of being seen within two weeks if certain criteria are met.
- A comprehensive assessment of their risk factors and angina.
- A full explanation and participation in planning of their management programme, which includes investigations such as exercise testing

and angiography, therapeutic interventions and lifestyle modifications.
• Regular review within primary care.

What this means for primary care teams

• Angina patients entered on primary care coronary heart disease registers.
• Primary healthcare teams offer programmes of structured care for angina patients.
• Local (PCO-wide) referral guidelines will need to be developed and implemented.
• An increase in investigation and revascularisation rates in the long term – the PCO will need to commission more services from the local cardiology unit. PCOs will be under pressure to divert resources to secondary care to fund manpower and equipment to meet the NSF standards.
• In the short term, primary care will be left to reconcile increasing patient expectations and generally poor access to secondary and tertiary care investigations and treatment.

Box 6.10 Tips

Primary care nurses should work with the cardiology liaison nurse at the local hospital to ensure:

• continuity of care following discharge and consistent messages to patients
• less duplication between primary and secondary care in managing secondary prevention
• common audit definitions, data and Read codes.

CHAPTER 7

Heart failure

> **Box 7.1** Standard 11 of the NSF
>
> Doctors should arrange for people with suspected heart failure to be offered appropriate investigations (e.g. echocardiography) that will confirm or refute the diagnosis. For those in whom heart failure is confirmed, its cause should be identified – the treatments most likely to both relieve symptoms and reduce their risk of death should be offered.

Heart failure is a common and deadly disease. However, the treatment and management of heart failure is a neglected area of under-rated importance. This is partly because the diagnosis of heart failure can be difficult. In general, there is too little good palliative care for those with heart failure.

Implementing the NSF will mean introducing the many effective interventions to as many patients with heart failure as possible via structured systematic care using disease registers and protocols that encompass primary, secondary and tertiary care.

Diagnosis

The NHS needs to improve diagnosis of heart failure, use of new therapies and structured systematic changes to remedy inappropriate primary care heart failure management.[36,67–69] The current situation is that misdiagnosis is common – people are labelled as having heart failure when their symptoms are due to other conditions (see below), and others with heart failure may be inadequately treated with the wrong drug or the wrong dose. Pathophysiologically, it can be defined as the inability of the heart to supply the circulatory needs of the body despite an adequate circulatory volume. The clinical definition (i.e. the recognition or diagnosis of heart failure) is not as straightforward. The symptoms consist of breathlessness, orthopnoea, fatigue and ankle swelling. The signs are a raised jugular venous pressure, crackles at the lung bases and peripheral oedema, and third or fourth heart sounds, tachycardia and a displaced apex beat.[13] Elevation of the jugular venous pressure and a displaced apex beat are the most specific signs, and may be difficult to elicit. The remaining clinical features can all be found with other conditions. Therefore misdiagnosis is common, both due to missing the diagnosis of heart failure and due to mislabelling of other diseases as heart failure.

As in all diagnoses, the context of the clinical findings is very important. For example, if a person was well before they suffered a myocardial infarction, and afterwards appears to have developed heart failure clinically, then no sophisticated tests are required, because there is little doubt that the clinical diagnosis will be correct.

Box 7.2 Simplified version of the New York Heart Association classification of heart failure symptoms[67]

Class I
No limitations – ordinary physical activity does not cause symptoms

Class II
Slight limitation of physical activity

Class III
Marked limitation of physical activity

Class IV
Inability to perform any physical activity without discomfort

---

The commonest cause of heart failure is coronary artery disease. Other causes include the following:

- hypertension
- valvular disease
- cor pulmonale
- cardiomyopathy (including idiopathic)
- drugs and alcohol.

Left ventricular hypertrophy, cigarette smoking, hyperlipidaemia and diabetes mellitus are all risk factors for heart failure.

Conditions which mimic heart failure include non-cardiac causes such as the following:

- drug-induced water retention (e.g. from non-steroidal anti-inflammatory drugs and calcium-channel blockers)
- physiological oedema in women
- renal disease
- liver disease
- pulmonary disease
- anaemia
- thyroid disease
- obesity
- bilateral renal artery stenosis.

Both the incidence and the prevalence of heart failure increase with age. The incidence of heart failure is difficult to estimate, and is thought to be around 0.1–0.4% of the population per year.[70] Heart failure is also more prevalent because the management of myocardial infarction has improved and more people survive for longer with subsequent heart failure. The prevalence of heart failure is 40 per 1000 men and 30 per 1000 women aged over 65 years, rising to 100 per 1000 for those over 80 years old.[13] It has been estimated that the prevalence of heart failure could increase by as much as 70% by the year 2010.[71]

Investigation of heart failure

There are around 6000 deaths a year due to heart failure associated with coronary heart disease. The six-year mortality rate of 80% is similar to that of many cancers.[67] The prognosis for moderate and severe heart failure is comparable to that of colorectal cancer, and worse than that of breast or prostate cancer.

Often, however, despite a structured and systematic approach to clinical assessment, accurate diagnosis requires further investigations.

The purpose of these investigations is to:

- confirm or exclude the diagnosis of heart failure
- define the precise underlying cause of heart failure if possible
- identify factors which alleviate or worsen the condition
- aid management and treatment decisions
- provide baseline information for future monitoring
- obtain prognostic information.

A diagnosis of heart failure is unlikely if there is nothing in the history or examination to suggest that there is anything wrong with the heart. Although that may seem so obvious as not to need stating, many such patients are mistakenly categorised as having heart failure. It is most important to identify a cause for the heart failure.

Routine blood investigations

These include the following:

- full blood count
- biochemical profile (urine and electrolytes, plasma/serum creatinine, liver enzymes, cholesterol and blood glucose)
- thyroid function tests.

Weight

A rapid gain in weight may indicate worsening heart failure, whilst weight loss may suggest over-diuresis.

Chest X-ray

Chest X-rays have a limited value in the diagnosis of heart failure. Cardiomegaly signifies the presence of heart disease but does not identify the cause of heart failure. Significant left ventricular dysfunction may occur in the absence of cardiomegaly. However, a chest X-ray will show cardiac enlargement, pulmonary venous congestion or pulmonary oedema.

ECG

Left ventricular dysfunction is very rare in the presence of a normal 12-lead ECG. However, an abnormal ECG does not mean that the patient has heart failure.

Echocardiography

This provides an accurate assessment of left ventricular systolic dysfunction and information on cardiac structure. It may also demonstrate features of diastolic dysfunction. Assessment of this is complex.

Radionuclide ventriculography

This provides the most accurate and reproducible assessment of left ventricular systolic dysfunction. Because of its expense and time-consuming nature it is not routinely indicated in the investigation of suspected heart failure.

Cost

Heart failure is an expensive condition to treat because of the high rates of hospital admission, and in fact it is the single commonest cause of hospital admission in the ÚK. Heart failure accounts for 5% of all adult medical admissions to hospital in the UK, and one-sixth of patients are readmitted with heart failure within six months of their first admission. The reasons for readmission include the following:

- uncontrolled symptoms
- non-adherence to medication
- non-compliance with diet (e.g. low salt)
- over-consumption of alcohol
- infection
- failed social support
- psychological problems.

What will implementing this NSF standard mean for patients?

It will mean:

- confirmation of the diagnosis by investigation if there is doubt
- a comprehensive assessment of their needs
- an individually tailored programme of care which includes lifestyle, therapeutic interventions and palliative care if appropriate
- access to specialist support as required (e.g. specialist smoking cessation clinics, dietary interventions and exercise programmes)
- arrangements for follow-up and review similar to other chronic disease management programmes, such as those for diabetes and asthma

- reduced hospital admission and readmission rates
- a better quality of palliative care
- improvements in the quality of life and in mortality.

The evidence for treatment of heart failure[13,47,70]

New developments in the drug treatment of heart failure include the potential addition of beta-blocker drugs or spironolactone to diuretic and ACE-inhibitor therapy. Angiotensin-II-receptor antagonists may be used as an alternative.

Angiotensin-converting-enzyme (ACE) inhibitors[72]

All patients with symptomatic heart failure and/or evidence of impaired left ventricular function should be treated with an ACE inhibitor. ACE inhibitors are associated with a 24% reduction in death rates in individuals with heart failure.[46]

Patients with a recent myocardial infarction and evidence of left ventricular dysfunction should be treated with an ACE inhibitor.

There is no evidence of any clinically important differences between ACE inhibitors, so patients should be treated with the cheapest ACE inhibitor that they can tolerate. It is critical that the recommended therapeutic doses are achieved.

ACE inhibitors can delay the development of symptomatic heart failure and reduce cardiovascular events in individuals with asymptomatic left ventricular systolic dysfunction and in people with other cardiovascular risk factors.

Angiotensin-II-receptor antagonists

None of these types of drugs is licensed in the UK for use in the treatment of heart failure. It is not clear whether they should be used instead of or in addition to an ACE inhibitor.[73]

The evidence supports the use of angiotensin-II-receptor blockers for patients who are truly intolerant of ACE inhibitors.[13]

Diuretics

Patients with signs of sodium and water retention (e.g. peripheral oedema) should receive diuretic therapy.

Adding ACE inhibitors to diuretics results in:[74]

- improved signs and symptoms of all grades of heart failure
- improved exercise tolerance
- slowing down of progression from mild to severe heart failure
- reduced hospital admission rates
- improved survival in all grades of heart failure
- enhanced functional status.

Patients who have already been treated with diuretics, an ACE inhibitor and/or digoxin, and who have moderate or severe heart failure (New York Heart Association classifications III and IV) should be considered for treatment with low-dose (25 mg) spironolactone. Adding spirono-lactone has been shown to decrease mortality and reduce the rate of hospital admissions.[13,72] Plasma/serum creatinine and electrolytes should be measured.

Beta-blocker drugs

Patients who have already been treated with diuretics and/or digoxin and an ACE inhibitor, who are clinically stable and in mild to moderate heart failure (New York Heart Association classification I–III) should be considered for treatment with a beta-blocker drug that is licensed for use in heart failure. Patients should initially be under specialist super-vision, as beta-blockers can make some patients with heart failure even more unwell. However, in view of the large numbers of patients involved, this level of specialist supervision may not be practicable, and local protocols should be developed. Overall, beta-blocker drugs reduce the risk of death by 36% compared with placebo.[75]

Recent evidence indicates that beta-blockers have an effect as great as, if not greater than, that of ACE inhibitors alone.[75] Most patients in these trials were already on ACE inhibitors. Thus the benefits of beta-blockers appear to be in addition to those derived from ACE inhibitors. Beta-blockers are most effective in patients with milder heart failure symptoms, and will slow down deterioration and increase the length of life as well as its quality.

Adding beta-blocker drugs to standard treatment with ACE inhibitors in patients with moderate heart failure reduces the rates of death and hospital admissions.[75] Around 74 patients with heart failure need to be treated with ACE inhibitors for one year to prevent one death, compared to 29 patients who need to be treated with beta-blocker drugs and only 21 patients who require treatment with both drugs in combination.

Currently, bisoprolol and carvedilol are licensed for use in the treatment of heart failure.

Beta-blocker drugs need to be started at a low dose that is then titrated up over a period of weeks or months. These drugs are also used in the treatment of patients with atrial fibrillation.

Digoxin

Digoxin has been shown to reduce the rate of hospital admissions, and co-intervention is recommended for worsening heart failure in patients who are already receiving diuretics and ACE inhibitors. There is no evidence that digoxin affects mortality.[13]

Digoxin is used for the following:

- all patients with heart failure and atrial fibrillation who need to have their ventricular rate controlled, and who cannot take beta-blocker drugs
- patients with moderately severe or severely symptomatic heart failure who remain symptomatic despite diuretic and ACE inhibitor therapy, or who have had more than one hospital admission for heart failure, or who have very poor left ventricular systolic function or persisting cardiomegaly
- patients with heart failure that have been treated with a diuretic, but who are unable to tolerate an ACE inhibitor or an angiotensin-II-receptor antagonist.

Patients who have already been treated with a diuretic and/or digoxin, but who are truly intolerant of an ACE inhibitor and angiotensin-II-receptor antagonist, should be considered for hydralazine and isosorbide dinitrate combination therapy.

Calcium-channel-blocker drugs

These drugs do not appear to have any benefit in patients with heart failure, and should be avoided.[13]

Anti-arrhythmic treatment

There is some inconclusive evidence that amiodarone reduces total mortality in patients with heart failure. However, other anti-arrhythmic drugs may increase mortality in patients with heart failure.[13]

Revascularisation/transplantation

Subgroups of heart failure patients may benefit from revascularisation/surgical transplantation.

Warfarin

Warfarin is used in cases of atrial fibrillation and heart failure.

Non-pharmacological and lifestyle measures for patients with heart failure

These can be summarised as follows.

1 Avoid salt-rich foods.
2 Offer an individualised exercise programme that is specifically tailored for heart failure if there are no contraindications.
3 Alcohol is contraindicated in alcohol-induced cardiomyopathy, but otherwise may be taken in small quantities (1–2 units per day).
4 Strategies for smoking cessation should be individually tailored.
5 Manage obesity with small stepped changes towards modest weight loss targets.
6 Cachexia should be dealt with by a physician and dietitian.

Home-based interventions

Heart failure frequently requires hospital admissions which are lengthy and expensive. A variety of studies have been undertaken to examine the effectiveness of non-pharmacological intervention programmes in the community setting that offer education and exercise, and promote therapeutic compliance and easy contact with professionals (nurse-led) if symptoms increase.

Empirically, patients with severe heart failure can often avoid the need for hospitalisation by weighing themselves daily, and receiving advice about treatment via the telephone. However, the results of trials are as yet inconclusive.

Continuing care

The management of heart failure in primary care should have a structured approach and include the following:

- risk factor advice, particularly relating to smoking cessation, physical activity, alcohol consumption and diet
- advice and treatment to control blood pressure
- immunisation annually against influenza and once for pneumo-coccus
- control of glucose levels and blood pressure in patients with diabetes
- assessment of social needs and provision of long-term support
- cardiac rehabilitation programmes
- palliative care.

Heart failure clinics[76]

Both the USA and Sweden favour nurse-led out-patient heart failure clinics. Such nurses have specialist education and training in heart failure, and they work to protocols developed by cardiologists.

It is important to understand the patient's beliefs about adherence to their prescribed medication and how the treatment affects their daily life. Educational interventions encompass the whole family. The educational programmes cover medical treatment and monitoring of symptoms. Lifestyle changes such as dietary adjustments, physical activity and infection prophylaxis are also included in the educational programmes. Management of symptoms is critical, and patients are taught to detect changes in their condition which may lead to a progression of heart failure (e.g. increasing shortness of breath, weight and/or oedema).

Palliative care

Good symptom control and psychological support should be offered to all patients. The aim should be to improve the quality of life by promoting physical, psychological and spiritual well-being. For those with advanced disease, specialist palliative care should be offered through multiprofessional teams. This is very rarely available for patients with heart failure at present.

Current practice

The majority of patients who are diagnosed with heart failure do not have echocardiography to determine whether they have left ventricular systolic dysfunction. In a study of 600 patients labelled as having heart failure, only 25% had definite left ventricular dysfunction. In total, 23 patients who had been labelled as having heart failure had atrial fibrillation, and most of those (60%) had normal left ventricular function. A further 20% had valvular abnormalities.[69]

The important issue of under-treatment and failure to use recommended doses of ACE inhibitors was illustrated in a Scottish study where it was found that 76% of heart failure patients were on maintenance doses lower than those used in major trials.[70] The initiative described in Box 7.3 below illustrates the multifaceted approach that is needed to improve prescribing and diagnostic accuracy of heart failure.

Box 7.3 Improving the management of heart failure

A multidisciplinary initiative in North Derbyshire improved the management of heart failure as measured by prescribing data for ACE inhibitors and diuretics, referrals for echocardiography, admissions and readmissions for heart failure, and hospital deaths from heart failure. The initiative included support for GPs and their practice teams to undertake an audit of their current practice in managing heart failure and in identifying patients with heart failure, an educational programme for patients with heart failure, and better access to diagnostic echocardiography. Prescribing of ACE inhibitors and loop diuretics increased by 18% and 27%, respectively, whilst prescribing of potassium-sparing diuretics decreased by 37% over a two-year period. Readmission and death rates in hospital from heart failure declined.[77]

Why is the management of heart failure suboptimal?

Most patients with heart failure initially present to their GP, but access to echocardiography is only available to a small proportion of GPs. In some parts of the country direct-access echocardiography services have been introduced, and this has led to the improvement in diagnosis of left ventricular systolic dysfunction.

The lack of prescribing of ACE inhibitors may be due to concerns about the potential adverse effects of ACE inhibitors. However, concerns about renal impairment and hypotension can be defused if creatinine is monitored appropriately and doses are tailored to the individual patient.

ECGs are more readily available than echocardiography, but interpretation is difficult in many cases.

What needs to be done to meet the NSF standard?

A structured approach is required for the management of heart failure patients.

1 Agree a protocol between general practice and the acute hospital with regard to the investigation and long-term management of heart failure patients.
2 Identify individuals with heart failure and create a heart failure register within general practice.
3 Establish a service which allows rapid access to echocardiography and/or cardiological opinion.
4 Offer a structured programme of care to patients with heart failure, including cardiac rehabilitation.
5 Make palliative care services available for end-stage heart failure.
6 Evaluate progress.

1 Developing a protocol

Protocols should include the following:

- arrangements for patient assessment and investigations – electrocardiography and echocardiography
- management arrangements, including general lifestyle interventions (e.g. smoking, patient support, dietary support and exercise programmes) and drug therapy
- arrangements for patient education and family support
- criteria for referral
- arrangements for continuing care and palliative care
- arrangements for follow-up.

The district protocol should cover the general practice and hospital settings.

2 Creating a heart failure register

The development of heart failure registers poses some difficult problems for primary care. This contrasts with the clear rationale for establishing CHD secondary prevention registers, as individuals with established angina and post-myocardial infarction can be defined relatively easily and identified without further secondary care-based investigations. Provision of structured care for CHD secondary prevention is a natural role for primary care nurses.

However, with regard to heart failure the diagnosis is uncertain in a large proportion of patients (up to 80%), and the services available to make diagnoses are deficient in many parts of the country where there is a lack of rapid access to echocardiography and expert specialist opinion. Primary care may not have the capacity to provide structured care with dedicated GP and nurse time for all those with a definitive diagnosis of heart failure. General practitioners may regard this area as too specialised for practice nurses to manage, because of the complexities surrounding diagnosis and management. This situation may change in the future as courses are established to help nurses to develop skills to provide structured care for heart failure.

Before embarking on the development of a heart failure register, consider the following questions.

- How will the diagnosis be established/confirmed?
- Will secondary care be able to cope with the increased demand for echocardiography and specialised cardiological opinion?
- Will primary care have sufficient capacity to review the diagnoses and management of these patients?

If the cardiology and investigative services are inadequate to deal with the management of patients with heart failure, then it is questionable whether heart failure disease registers should be established.

There needs to be clear rationale for the establishment of registers.

- Is it to review the management of these patients by establishing a diagnosis and developing a management plan, and then delivering this service?
- Is it just to monitor the progress of these patients for audit purposes?
- Or is it for both reasons?

Who should be included on a heart failure register?

Possible approaches include the following.

Newly diagnosed patients

If only newly diagnosed patients with a definitive diagnosis of heart failure are included on the register, they could be provided with the optimum treatment. There would be a minimal impact on primary and secondary services, as the numbers would be relatively small. However, this approach would be inequitable.

Newly diagnosed and existing patients with a clear diagnosis of heart failure

If only this group were to be included on the heart failure disease register, this would have a limited impact on secondary care services, as presumably most of these patients will either have had an echocardiogram already or have a clear clinical diagnosis. However, there will be significant numbers of patients for primary care to review and follow up.

All patients labelled as having heart failure within primary care where the diagnosis of heart failure is not necessarily supported by clear diagnostic evidence

Establishing a diagnosis in these patients will take up considerable resources in primary care and hospital services. It will also present the challenge of deciding who should be reviewed first. Echocardiography will not only provide information about the structural defects of the heart, but will also aid the development of a management plan for patients.

Some very difficult choices will need to be made, as heart failure patients consume a considerable amount of NHS resources because of the very high rate of readmission to hospital. Should patients who are currently admitted and frequently readmitted through a revolving door between primary and secondary care be prioritised for structured care at the expense of newly diagnosed patients with a clear diagnosis?

Opportunistic approach

An alternative approach is to establish a heart failure disease register on a 'first come, first served' basis (i.e. patients – irrespective of diagnostic certainty – are entered on a register as they come into contact with primary care). Patients are then offered an opportunity to establish a definitive diagnosis if necessary and a comprehensive programme of structured care. The advantage of this approach is that difficult priority decisions can be avoided and the register is developed over a period of time.

Box 7.4 describes how primary care groups in one locality are tackling the identification and management of patients with heart failure.

Box 7.4 Setting up a heart failure register across a primary care organisation

The following groups of patients should be clinically examined and reviewed:

1 patients who have a recorded diagnosis of heart failure on existing databases (e.g. CHD and diabetes registers)
2 patients who have had echocardiograms where a diagnosis of heart failure was made
3 patients who have been prescribed loop diuretics within the last six months
4 patients who have been prescribed ACE inhibitors, excluding those with a diagnosis of hypertension
5 patients who have been prescribed digoxin or any other cardiac glycoside.

In addition, scrutinise patients who are seen opportunistically.

Categorisation of patients at clinical review

Patients should be allocated into one of the following three groups after being reviewed:

---

1 patients who have proven heart failure or a very high clinical suspicion of heart failure
2 patients who are likely to have heart failure but who would benefit from further investigation in the future, should the clinical need arise
3 patients who are unlikely to have heart failure

Creating the register

Patients allocated to groups 1 and 2 after clinical review should be recorded on the practice's clinical computer system with the appropriate Read code (G58) as having heart failure. This group will then become the register. Record whether the patient has had an echocardiogram and whether this is normal or abnormal.

Secondary care services would find it difficult to cope with demand if all of the patients identified in category 2 were referred for an echocardiogram to confirm the diagnosis. Therefore these patients should only be referred if the clinical need arises. Identify those patients in group 2 with a specific Read code or keep a separate list of patients manually. Patients allocated to group 3 should have all references to heart failure removed from their summary record in order to avoid their inclusion in any future interrogation of the data.

Keep an accurate record of all comorbidity in patients on the register.

Coding

The Read code G58 for heart failure is the main stem code. The record of echocardiography in such patients when this investigation has been performed should be entered as follows:

echocardiogram normal – 58530
echocardiogram abnormal – 58531.

(Adapted from Lichfield, Burntwood and Tamworth Primary Care Groups.)

3 Access to echocardiography

Increased access to echocardiography will be essential to improve the accuracy of diagnoses and the quality of management plans. A variety of options exist for local services, ranging from direct access to echocardiography, to referral to secondary care heart failure clinics.

Box 7.5

In a recent study,[78] 126 patients with a clinical diagnosis of heart failure were examined by echocardiogram. The investigators found that:

- reliance on ECG alone avoided 60 of 120 echocardiograms, at the cost of missing one patient with left ventricular systolic dysfunction
- if an echocardiogram was performed only in patients with an abnormal ECG and either increased atrial natriuretic peptide or a heart rate greater than the diastolic pressure, then 100 out of 120 tests were avoided at the cost of missing the diagnosis in four patients.

4 Providing a structured programme of care within primary care

Models of care range from a focus on specialist care in the hospital setting to good routine care in GP consultations.

- Heart failure clinics within the hospital setting could either investigate and follow up patients, or initiate treatments and refer patients to primary care for further management. Specialist nurses based in hospital can provide an outreach service both for patients admitted to hospital and after their discharge, and facilitate training and development of services within the primary care setting – a similar approach to that adopted by diabetes specialist nurses.
- Multidisciplinary teams manage patients with established heart failure in the primary care setting. These might include input from the specialist nurse, local pharmacists, palliative care nurses, social carers and dietitians, as well as members of the core primary healthcare team.
- Patients with heart failure could be managed in general practice nurse-led cardiovascular secondary prevention clinics. Primary care nurses operate within agreed protocols that include their development and training to manage the long-term care of patients with heart failure.
- Review of patients could take place within normal GP consultations. Patients are systematically invited from the register to attend for regular assessment and management, with longer consultation times allotted.

5 Palliative care service for patients with end-stage heart failure

GPs and other health professionals should be well informed about the full range of palliative care services for end-stage heart failure, and they should know how to help patients to access such help.

6 Evaluation

Consider how well you are faring against the milestones stated in the NSF.[2] For example, do you have a protocol describing the systematic assessment, treatment and follow-up of patients with heart failure? To what extent do you provide structured care in line with the protocol (use audit to find out, and also ask patients themselves).

The goal in the NSF against which you should be auditing your care is that 'every primary care team should ensure that all those with heart failure are receiving a full package of appropriate investigations and treatments, demonstrated by clinical audit no more than 12 months old.'

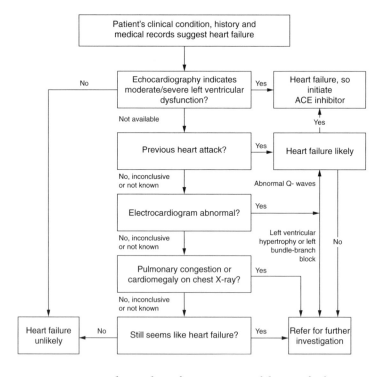

Figure 7.1: Diagnostic algorithm for suspected heart failure in primary care (modified from North of England Evidence-Based Guideline Development Project[54]).

Roles and responsibilities of the primary healthcare team

These suggestions are just ideas and are not intended to be comprehensive.

Primary care organisations (PCOs)

The PCO's responsibilities include leadership, assisting primary care teams to develop registers, identifying training needs and provision of training support, developing services to meet local needs (e.g. open-access echocardiography) and supporting clinical audit.

Leadership

Roles and responsibilities include the following:

- assessing local needs of heart failure patients
- raising the profile of heart failure patients through workshops, etc.
- understanding and communicating the projected increase in the number of heart failure patients, the evidence base for best practice and the health economics of heart failure
- reaching a local consensus on models for a heart failure service to meet local needs.

Supporting the development of a heart failure register

1 Identify people with heart failure.
    - Agree definitions, including standard Read codes, across the PCO (*see* Appendix 1).
    - Assist practices in computerised searching for patients with heart failure (e.g. by using drug names, Read codes, practitioners' personal knowledge, or hospital lists of patients admitted with heart failure).
    - Support practices in validating the notes to ensure that patients are correctly identified.
2 Develop a template.
    - Develop a PCO-wide consensus on the template to be used.
    - Ensure that the template is incorporated into various IT systems.

- Support the practices in integrating the template into practice software.
- Provide technical IT support when problems arise.
- Provide technical IT support when practices change computer systems.

3 Enter data into computer databases.
- Provide options for resourcing data entry.
- Support practices in validating data entry.
- Ensure that practices have arrangements for entering new patients.
- Ensure that practices have systems to maintain registers, and that primary care team members are committed to this as a long-term project.

Assessing the training needs of primary care teams

The PCO will need to have an overview of training needs within primary care teams throughout the constituency in order to achieve the right balance between specialist and core work.

Developing local services

Undertake a needs assessment, and enlist the help of the local public health department. The needs assessment should include the following:

- incidence of heart failure
- prevalence of heart failure
- mortality due to heart failure
- evidence of the effectiveness of interventions
- description of current services, including diagnostic services, prescribing patterns and current management
- views of local professionals
- views of users and voluntary groups
- development of an ideal model
- the gap between current provision and the ideal model
- costing of services
- an action plan for change.

A case for an open-access echocardiography service or an out-patient heart failure clinic could be made by undertaking a needs assessment.

Supporting clinical audit and evaluation of services

Set your criteria for evaluating current services to include indicators that can be measured over time to show the effects of your action plan and subsequent changes. As in the example from North Derbyshire cited in Box 7.3, the indicators might include the following:

- ACE and diuretic prescribing rates
- length of hospital stay for heart failure
- hospital admission and readmission rates
- death rates.

GPs

- Take ultimate responsibility for the way in which the practice identifies patients with heart failure, sets up practice registers, and validates the diagnosis of patients classified as having heart failure on the disease register.
- Agree practice protocols with the PCO and practice team.
- Invest in the team providing care for patients with heart failure and equipment to be able to provide best practice.
- Know and undertake your own roles and responsibilities with regard to preventing and managing heart failure – according to the agreed protocols.

Primary care nurses

- Help with the identification of patients with heart failure from personal contacts or by searching notes.
- Contribute to designing the practice protocol for the management of heart failure.
- Incorporate the identification and management of heart failure in ongoing secondary prevention CHD clinics.
- Link with other nurses within the PCO or the hospital to provide specialist care.
- Evaluate changes resulting from new initiatives within the primary care setting (e.g through audits).
- Identify your own learning needs, and feed these back to practice managers or via clinical supervision to aid the organisation of appropriate education and training.

Practice managers

- Know the milestones and standards expected by the NSF for coronary heart disease.

- Liaise with the PCO over the implementation of those milestones and standards.
- Organise the systems and structures in the practices to be able to identify patients with heart failure, set up disease registers, undertake audit, and provide best practice in managing heart failure.

Pharmacists

- Be up to date on the management of heart failure, in order to be able to answer customers' questions and reinforce best practice.
- Help with the identification of patients with heart failure if asked by local practices (e.g. from medication records).
- Contribute to the drawing up of practice protocols to ensure that the role of the pharmacist is incorporated.

Patients

- Adhere to the treatment prescribed by the GP which conforms to best practice – after the purpose has been explained and an individual treatment plan negotiated.
- Report any intolerance of drugs, and work with the GP to find suitable alternatives, rather than stop taking the medication.
- Adopt as well balanced a lifestyle (e.g. diet, exercise non-smoking, etc.) as personal circumstances permit.

Box 7.6 Tips for combating heart failure

A normal ECG and chest X-ray will virtually exclude the diagnosis of heart failure.

Strategies for identifying heart failure patients include the following:

1 identifying newly presenting and old patients discharged from hospital with a label of heart failure/left ventricular dysfunction
2 screening opportunistically through diabetic, hypertension and CHD secondary prevention clinics for patients with heart failure
3 undertaking search strategies for patients on diuretic and ACE-inhibitor drugs. However, most of these patients will have hypertension, and you will have to be careful to select only those with heart failure. This approach will be time-consuming.

CHAPTER 8

Cardiac rehabilitation

Box 8.1 Standard 12 of the NSF

The NHS trust should put in place agreed protocols/systems of care so that, prior to leaving hospital, people admitted to hospital suffering from coronary heart disease have been invited to participate in a multidisciplinary programme of secondary prevention and cardiac rehabilitation.

Patients who have been admitted to hospital because of a myocardial infarction are among those at greatest risk of further cardiac events and death. Cardiac rehabilitation should reduce the risk of subsequent cardiac problems and promote a return to a full and normal life.

Like all major illnesses, cardiac disease has physical, psychological and behavioural components, and there is a complex interaction between the patient's recovery and social and family influences. The psychological consequences of myocardial infarction can be more disabling than the physical state. They can also dictate the extent to which the patient responds to the various interventions and converts to a healthy lifestyle.

Box 8.2 Delivering community-based cardiac rehabilitation through a *Heart Manual*

The *Heart Manual* is produced by Edinburgh Health Care Trust, and is a six-week community-based programme delivering rehabilitation. The scheme can be administered by health visitors, and the patient-held *Heart Manual* answers commonly asked questions about medicines and lifestyle, as well as providing a structured programme based on simple exercises.[79]

Cardiac rehabilitation aims to help patients to regain their confidence so that they can enjoy the best possible physical, mental and emotional health. It should be an intrinsic part of the management of all types of cardiac disease. Programmes of cardiac rehabilitation should be specifically tailored to an individual's needs – including education, psychological interventions and exercise activities.

Although cardiac rehabilitation has been targeted at patients who have had a myocardial infarction or who have undergone coronary artery bypass surgery in the past, patients with stable angina and those with heart failure can benefit, too.[80]

Cardiac rehabilitation phases

These are as follows:

- phase 1 – in-hospital interventions before discharge
- phase 2 – immediate post-discharge period
- phase 3 – four weeks after an acute cardiac invent
- phase 4 – long-term maintenance of changed behaviour.

Components of cardiac rehabilitation

Cardiac rehabilitation includes the following:

- exercise
- psychosocial interventions
- education
- therapeutic interventions.

Patients who benefit from cardiac rehabilitation include the following:

- those who are post-acute myocardial infarction
- before and after revascularisation procedures
- those with stable angina
- those with heart failure
- cases associated with other specialised interventions, such as cardiac transplant.

Benefits for patients

Patients can expect the following:

- provision of skilled help and individually tailored programmes of care
- help with understanding their illness and its treatment
- psychological and emotional support
- practical support in making healthy lifestyle choices
- help with making the transition back to normal life activities
- a reduced risk of heart attack and death from cardiac events.

Box 8.3 Home-based cardiac rehabilitation[27]

A surgery in Cornwall offers home-based rehabilitation for those who have suffered and survived a heart attack. The cardiac rehabilitation programme is centred around the *Heart Manual*. Following the heart attack, patients are assessed in order to determine their suitability for entry to the home-based rehabilitation programme, which is closely linked with the hospital-based rehabilitation team.

Contact: Lower Lemon Street Surgery, Truro. Tel: 01872 273 133.

Comparison of current service provision and uptake

Despite the evidence for its effectiveness, only a small proportion of patients who could benefit from cardiac rehabilitation complete a full cardiac rehabilitation programme, and less than half of the 150 000 individuals who survive a heart attack each year receive any form of rehabilitation. Particularly low uptake rates can be found in disadvantaged social groups such as ethnic minorities, and among women in general.[80] Other people with low uptake and special needs include those on low incomes, elderly people, individuals with physical disability, and those who live a long distance from a specialist cardiology unit.

Implications for primary care

- Patients who are suitable for cardiac rehabilitation also need to be entered into general practice secondary prevention CHD programmes and provided with associated support (e.g. nurse-led secondary prevention clinics, smoking cessation clinics).
- There are opportunities to develop community-based cardiac rehabilitation schemes (e.g. through partnership with leisure services or primary care-based schemes).

CHAPTER 9

Atrial fibrillation

A hospital-based study estimated the prevalence of atrial fibrillation to be around 2.5% of the population, which makes it the most commonly encountered cardiac arrhythmia. Prevalence increases with age, and about 10% of people in their eighties have atrial fibrillation.

Atrial fibrillation is a very strong risk factor for stroke. There have been five large randomised primary prevention trials which have demonstrated that anticoagulation with warfarin reduces the risk of stroke by 68%, compared with a 21% reduction in those using aspirin. For those patients who have had a stroke, anticoagulation also reduces the risk of further strokes (i.e. as part of secondary prevention).[13]

The risk of intracranial haemorrhage increases with anticoagulation, and the evidence seems to suggest that the optimum international normalised ratio (INR) for anticoagulation in non-valvular atrial fibrillation should be between 2.0 and 3.0. This target should minimise the risk of intracranial haemorrhage whilst providing maximal thromboprophylaxis.[13,81]

Elderly people (i.e. those over 75 years of age) are at high risk of the complications of atrial fibrillation, and the risk of stroke is also highest in this age group.[82] Anticoagulants should be prescribed on an individual case basis.

Near-patient testing

Computerised support systems and near-patient testing schemes are being introduced to facilitate primary care-based anticoagulation monitoring.

Other anti-thrombotic agents

There is little evidence to support the use of dipyridamole, clopidogrel and ticlopidine as a substitute for warfarin in the prevention of stroke in patients with atrial fibrillation. Aspirin may be suitable in low-risk patients with atrial fibrillation, but the optimum dosage is not clear.

Assessment of risk

The risk of stroke resulting from non-valvular atrial fibrillation is about 5% per year. Patients who are at highest risk of stroke include those over 75 years of age who have other risks factors, such as:

- diabetes
- hypertension
- past history of transient ischaemic attack or stroke
- valve disease
- heart failure
- thyroid disease.

Patients at moderate risk include those under 65 years of age with risk factors such as hypertension and diabetes. Also at moderate risk are those above the age of 65 years who do not have any of the high-risk factors.

People at low risk of stroke include those under the age of 65 years with no history of embolism, hypertension, diabetes or other clinical risk factors. These individuals have an annual risk of stroke of 1% or less.

Treatment

- *High risk*: use warfarin (target INR in the range 2.0–3.0).
- *Moderate risk*: use aspirin or warfarin. Aspirin is recommended for high- or moderate-risk patients who decline warfarin or who are poor candidates for warfarin.
- *Low risk*: use aspirin (75–300 mg once daily).

How current practice compares with the evidence

The use of anticoagulation for patients with atrial fibrillation is uncommon in the UK. In one study in the UK, only 76% of patients had the diagnosis recorded in their GP notes, and in another community survey only 30% of patients with atrial fibrillation had ever presented to hospital practice.[26,83]

The reasons for infrequent use of anticoagulation include the following:

- GP concerns about the safety of anticoagulation, in particular the risk of cerebral haemorrhage, especially in the elderly
- difficulties in long-term monitoring of the INR
- patients who are reluctant to attend busy hospital clinics on a regular basis
- increased workload for GPs who manage warfarin anticoagulation in primary care.

Implications for primary care

- Adopt evidence-based guidelines for the management of atrial fibrillation.
- Anticipate the increased workload involved in identifying suitable patients, establishing atrial fibrillation registers, confirming the diagnosis, establishing the cause of atrial fibrillation, explaining the risks and benefits of anti-coagulation to patients, and developing monitoring and review arrangements.
- Explore the alternatives for anticoagulant monitoring (e.g. via the hospital clinic, pharmacist-led monitoring arrangements, primary care clinic, GP clinics shared between practices).

CHAPTER 10

Using personal development plans and practice personal and professional development plans to improve the quality of coronary heart disease care and services provided

If we are to provide uniformly high-quality care and services for coronary heart disease, then health professionals should approach their continuing professional development in a more systematic way, too, rather than in the *ad-hoc* manner that has been usual in the past. We should be moving towards team-based learning that includes everyone, whether they are a doctor, nurse, therapist, manager or non-clinical worker. Attached nursing and therapy staff, and other independent contractors (e.g. community pharmacists) should be drawn into practice educational plans as they evolve.

Individual personal development plans should tie in with practice-based personal and professional development plans. These in turn are linked with those of their primary care organisation (PCO). The plans will underpin the revalidation of clinicians' professional registration or the accreditation of practices and PCOs in the future.[3]

The future lies in multidisciplinary learning together as practice teams. Individual practices will contribute to a coherent plan for their PCO's population to provide healthcare that is relevant to local needs. Practice personal and professional development plans will be a vehicle for the clinical governance programme, taking forward the objectives in the practice's or PCO's business and development plans.[5]

Practice-based educational plans should equip the practice team members to:

- minimise inequalities in the health of different subgroups of the population
- reduce variations in the standards and range of healthcare services
- define standards for multidisciplinary delivery of care and services
- demonstrate achievements
- sustain quality improvements.

You may decide to allocate 50% of the time you intend to spend drawing up and applying a personal development plan in any one year to learning more about coronary heart disease. That would leave space in your learning plan for other important topics such as diabetes, mental health care or cancer – whatever is a priority for you, the practice team and your patient population. There will be some overlap between topics – you cannot consider a person with coronary heart disease in isolation from their mental health and general well-being.

You might start by asking everyone to identify their own learning needs, and then combining them with those of other people and checking them against the practice business plan. Alternatively, you could start from the opposite direction, by developing a practice-based personal and professional development plan from your business plan and then identifying everyone's individual learning needs within that. Whichever direction you start from, you must ensure that you integrate team members' individual needs with those of your practice and with the needs and directives of the NHS.

Make your learning plan flexible. You may want to add something later when circumstances suddenly change or an additional need becomes apparent, perhaps as a result of a complaint, the launch of a new drug or new requirements issued by the government, the PCO or the National Institute for Clinical Excellence (NICE).

Long-term locums (e.g. longer than six months), assistants, retained doctors and salaried GPs should all be included in the practice plan. Remember to include all those staff who work for the practice, however few their hours – you cannot manage without them or they would not be there!

Time is one of the resources that must be considered when drawing up your action plan. Adequate resources must be in place for your learning needs, and protected time must be built in.

Read through the worked examples – they are just a simple guide to how you might start. There is a brief version of a personal development plan focusing on smoking cessation, and a brief version of a practice personal and professional development plan focusing on coronary heart disease in general. If you want to look at examples of personal development plans and practice personal and professional development plans in more detail look at other related publications.

Wakley G, Chambers R and Field S (2000) *Continuing Professional Development in Primary Care: making it happen.* Radcliffe Medical Press, Oxford.

Chambers R, Wakley G and Iqbal Z (2001) *Cardiovascular Disease Matters in Primary Care.* Radcliffe Medical Press, Oxford.

Abbreviated worked example: personal development plan focusing on smoking cessation

This topic is a priority for learning because you will want to implement the most cost-effective ways of delivering smoking cessation in the practice. Smoking cessation is a priority in the National Service Framework for Coronary Heart Disease (for England).

Learning needs

These can be identified by, for example:

- running an audit on the practice computer to see how many patients are registered as current smokers
- undertaking an audit to find out how many of the patients you have advised to stop smoking in the past have actually stopped
- reading about smoking cessation in a compendium of evidence such as Barton S (2000) *Clinical Evidence.* Issue 4. BMJ Publishing Group, London. How much did you know already and how much do you still have to learn?
- completing a SWOT analysis of strengths, weaknesses, opportunities and threats with regard to smoking cessation from your own personal perspectives and those of your practice at a practice team meeting or with a trusted colleague.

Patient or public input to your personal development plan: consult your practice's patient participation group if you have one about how you might run the smoking cessation service so that it is convenient for patients. Alternatively, hold a roadshow in the practice one evening on the subject of stopping smoking, advertise it widely and invite suggestions as to how you might improve your care and services.

Aim of your personal development plan arising from the preliminary data-gathering exercise: to find out which interventions reduce cigarette smoking most effectively and to apply those interventions in practice (resources permitting).

Integrate the 14 components of clinical governance into your personal development plan focusing on smoking cessation: look back at Chapter 1 for ideas on how you might do this.

Action plan in brief – an example

By 2 months

Preliminary data have been gathered:

- skills that you already have
- equipment and systems that are available (yours and those of the practice, the PCO, and outside in a training venue)
- training that can be obtained (to match your needs)
- identify learning needs (see above).

By 4 months

Review current performance:
- review the results of audits of how well you are able to motivate patients to change their behaviour and stop smoking
- review the number of patients whose smoking status you know (is data recorded consistently by you or other colleagues?)
- look at the opportunities arising from your SWOT analysis.

By 6 months

Identify solutions to your learning needs:

- arrange the necessary training, with cover
- make a business plan for any associated equipment needs
- clarify who does what, and when, in your practice protocol
- attend learning activities; read and reflect.

By 12 months

Make the changes and put your learning into practice:

- implement the new systems or procedures
- obtain feedback from patients and other staff about its impact
- identify any further gaps in your knowledge and skills, and the provision of services.

Expected outcomes

An increasing proportion of patients (set the exact target depending on your current baseline) with established heart disease, and those at risk of heart disease, have their smoking status recorded. Smokers receive effective 'stop-smoking' advice. Those who are ready to do so receive smoking cessation therapy based on the best evidence of what works.

Evaluating the personal development plan: set specific objectives before starting, and compare against these at timed intervals the progress that you are making. Evaluate whether the type of learning activities you chose to follow were the most appropriate for what you aimed to learn. Evaluate the extent to which your new learning is applied in practice.

Keep a record of your learning and reflection: this should include both formal and informal, in-house and external learning activities.

Abbreviated worked example: practice personal and professional development plan focusing on coronary heart disease

This topic is a priority for learning because, for example, the practice team undertook a significant event audit after the unexpected death of a 45-year-old from a myocardial infarction. CHD is a national priority, and is the subject of a National Service Framework.

Who will be included in the practice personal and professional development plan?

- GPs
- practice nurses

- practice manager
- receptionists
- district nurses
- community pharmacists
- health visitors
- public and patients.

Learning needs

These could be identified by you as a practice collecting information about the following:

- all recent practice-based initiatives (e.g. suggestions from patients/ staff, minutes of practice meetings during the last 12 months which are relevant)
- any recent audit of the extent of aspirin-taking by those for whom it is clinically warranted with regard to their history of CHD
- practice-based prescribing data on statins, hypertensive drugs and aspirin
- the health profile of the local community, local morbidity and mortality rates from the health authority (compare any practice-specific data with district figures)
- the health improvement programme and other relevant district health reports and strategies (How relevant do they seem to your circumstances? What can you learn from them to help you in your everyday work?)
- district guidelines on referrals to the cardiology directorate – compare your referral patterns with those advised
- published guidelines on the management of cardiac conditions and hypertension – compare your practice protocols and see whether you can justify any variations.

Patient or public input to your practice learning plan: you might target patients who do not attend or who do not adhere to recommended treatment, and find out why by asking them directly.

How will you prioritise everyone's needs in a fair and open way? A practice meeting might be devoted to this question.

Aim of the practice personal and professional development plan arising from the preliminary data-gathering exercise: to develop a learning programme that underpins the timed achievement of milestones within the standards of the National Service Framework on coronary heart disease.

Integrate the 14 components of clinical governance into your practice personal and professional development plan focusing on CHD: look back at Chapter 1 for ideas on how you might do this.

Action plan in brief

By 3 months

Preliminary data gathering and collation of baseline:

- are there practice protocols for the management of the various components of CHD?
- map the numbers of staff, map expertise and list other providers
- review referral patterns for CHD conditions (acute admissions and routine)
- obtain information about the characteristics of those recorded on the practice computer as having CHD.

By 5 months

Review current performance:

- practice manager reviews operation of services and links with other organisations and sectors with an interest in or responsibility for CHD (e.g. cardiac rehabilitation)
- clinical lead reviews the extent of the knowledge and skills of the practice team with regard to routine care of all aspects of CHD
- audit actual performance vs. pre-agreed criteria for various topics
- compare performance with any or several of the 14 components of clinical governance (e.g. clinical risk management would be very relevant).

By 6 months

Identify solutions and associated training needs:

- set up new systems for access to services appropriate to people's needs
- give the practice team in-house training and arrange external courses
- revise practice protocols.

By 12 months

Make changes:

- clinicians adhere to practice protocol for CHD, as shown by repeat audits
- establish secondary prevention clinics run by a trained practice nurse and GP with a special interest in CHD
- change the service times and locations to ones that are more appropriate for patients with CHD or who are at risk. Organise training to anticipate new requirements.

Expected outcomes

These include more effective prevention of CHD in general, better compliance with treatment and healthy lifestyle advice, revised practice protocols for the management of hypertension, control of hyperlipidaemia, and ultimately lives saved.

Evaluating the practice personal and professional development plan: the practice might re-audit their management of hypertension, hyper-lipidaemia and post-myocardial infarction one year after embarking on the plan. There might be observation of practice, review of achievements during subsequent educational or job appraisals, or a repeat computer search to check developments with the CHD register.

Keep a record of your learning and reflection: this should include both formal and informal, in-house and external learning activities.

References

1 Secretary of State for Health (1999) *Saving Lives: our healthier nation.* Department of Health, London.
2 NHS Executive (2000) *National Service Framework for Coronary Heart Disease.* Department of Health, London.
3 Wakley G, Chambers R and Field S (2000) *Continuing Professional Development: making it happen.* Radcliffe Medical Press, Oxford.
4 Lilley R (1999) *Making Sense of Clinical Governance.* Radcliffe Medical Press, Oxford.
5 Chambers R and Wakley G (2000) *Making Clinical Governance Work for you.* Radcliffe Medical Press, Oxford.
6 Mohanna K and Chambers R (2001) *Risk Matters: communicating risk, clinical risk management.* Radcliffe Medical Press, Oxford.
7 Commission for Health Improvement (2001) *Training Manual for Review Team Members.* Commission for Health Improvement, London.
8 Miller C, Ross N and Freeman M (1999) *Shared Learning and Clinical Teamwork: new directions in education and multiprofessional practice.* English National Board for Nursing, Midwifery and Health Visiting, University of Brighton, Brighton.
9 Chambers R (2000) *Involving Patients and the Public. How to do it better.* Radcliffe Medical Press, Oxford.
10 Hofman A and Vandenbroucke JP (1992) Geoffrey Rose's big idea. Changing the population distribution of a risk factor is better than targeting people at high-risk. *BMJ.* **305**: 1519–20.
11 Department of Health (1997) Report of the review of patient-identifiable information. In: *The Caldicott Committee Report.* Department of Health, London.
12 Muir Gray JA (1997) *Evidence-Based Healthcare.* Churchill Livingstone, Edinburgh.
13 Barton S (ed.) (2001) *Clinical Evidence.* Issue 5. BMJ Publishing Group, London.
14 Royal College of General Practitioners (Scotland), Scottish Heart and Arterial Disease Risk Prevention, and Scottish Intercollegiate Guidelines Network (2000) *The Heart Pack: coronary heart disease resource directory.* Royal College of General Practitioners, Edinburgh.
15 Scottish Intercollegiate Guidelines Network (1999) *Lipids and the Primary Prevention of Coronary Heart Disease.* Scottish Intercollegiate Guidelines Network Secretariat, Edinburgh.

16 Scottish Intercollegiate Guidelines Network (2000) *Secondary Prevention of Coronary Heart Disease Following Myocardial Infarction.* Scottish Intercollegiate Guidelines Network Secretariat, Edinburgh.

17 Department of Health (2000) *Statistics on Smoking Cessation Services in Health Action Zones: England, April 1999 to March 2000.* Statistical Press Release. Department of Health, London.

18 Irvine D and Irvine S (1991) *Making Sense of Audit.* Radcliffe Medical Press, Oxford.

19 NHS Executive (2000) *The NHS Plan.* NHS Executive, London.

20 Ebrahim S, Davey-Smith G, McCabe C *et al.* (1999) What role for statins? A review and economic model. A review. *Health Technol Assess.* **3**: 1–91.

21 National Heart Forum (1999) *Looking to the Future: making coronary heart disease an epidemic of the past.* The Stationery Office, London.

22 Doctor Awards (2000) Dr Peter Tyerman and Practice Team, Barnsley, Yorkshire. Coronary Heart Disease category. Reed Healthcare Publishing, Sutton.

23 Primatesta P and Poulter N (2000) Lipid concentrations and the use of lipid-lowering drugs: evidence from a national cross-sectional survey. *BMJ.* **321**: 1322–5.

24 Monkman D (2000) Treating dyslipidaemia in primary care. *BMJ.* **321**: 1299–300.

25 Moore A and McQuay H (eds) (2000) Better health through better lifestyle. *Bandolier.* **7**: 3–4.

26 Smith C and Pratt M (1993) Cardiovascular disease. In: *Chronic Disease Epidemiology and Control.* American Public Health Association, Washington, DC.

27 NHS Beacon Services (2000) *NHS Beacons Learning Handbook 2000/ 2001.* Volume 1. NHS Beacon Services, Petersfield.

28 Oliver M (1991) Might treatment of hypercholesterolaemia increase non-cardiac mortality? *Lancet.* **337**: 1529–31.

29 Office for National Statistics (2000) *Drug Use, Smoking and Drinking Among Teenagers in 1999.* Office for National Statistics, London.

30 Secretary of State for Health and Secretaries of State for Scotland, Wales and Northern Ireland (1998) *Smoking Kills: a White Paper on tobacco.* The Stationery Office, London.

31 Office for National Statistics (2000) *Living in Britain: results from the 1998 General Household Survey.* The Stationery Office, London.

32 Godfrey C, Raw M, Sutton M *et al.* (1993) *The Smoking Epidemic: a prescription for change.* Health Education Authority, London.

33 Action on Smoking and Health (ASH) (2000) *Basic Facts No 1: smoking statistics, January 2000.* Action on Smoking and Health, London.

34 Peto R, Darby S, Deo H *et al.* (2000) Smoking, smoking cessation, and lung cancer in the UK since 1950: combination of national statistics with two case–control studies. *BMJ.* **321**: 323–9.

35 Fowler G (2000) Smoking cessation: a key role for primary care. *Update.* **May**: 3–8.

36 Lancaster T, Stead L, Silagy C and Sowden A for Cochrane Tobacco Addiction Review Group (2000) Effectiveness of interventions to help people stop smoking: findings from the Cochrane Library. *BMJ.* **321**: 355–8.

37 Tobacco Advisory Group (2000) *Nicotine Addiction in Britain.* Royal College of Physicians, London.

38 Collier J (ed.) (2000) Bupropion to aid smoking cessation. *Drug Ther. Bull.* **38**: 73–5.

39 Fowler G (2000) Helping smokers to stop: an evidence-based approach. *Practitioner.* **244**: 37–41.

40 Sivers F (1999) *Evidence-Based Strategies for Secondary Prevention of Coronary Heart Disease* (2e). A and M Publishing, Guildford.

41 Reference Family Health Study Group (1994) RCT evaluating cardiovascular screening and intervention in general practice: principles of the British Family Heart Study. *BMJ.* **308**: 313–20.

42 OXCHECK Study Group (1995) Effectiveness of health checks conducted by nurses in primary care; final results of the OXCHECK Study. *BMJ.* **310**: 99–104.

43 Antiplatelet Trialists' Collaboration (1994) Collaborative overview of randomised trials of antiplatelet therapy. 1. Prevention of death, myocardial infarction and stroke by prolonged antiplatelet therapy in various categories of patients. *BMJ.* **308**: 81–106.

44 Scandinavian Simvastatin Survival Study Group (1995) Randomised trial of cholesterol lowering in 4444 patients with coronary heart disease: the Scandinavian Simvastatin Survival Study (4S). *Lancet.* **344**: 1383–9.

45 Long-term Intervention with Pravastatin in Ischaemic Disease (LIPID) Study Program (1998) Prevention of cardiovascular events and death with pravastatin in patients with coronary heart disease and a broad range of initial cholesterol levels. *NEJM.* **339**: 1349–57.

46 Sacks FM, Pfeffer MA, Moye LA *et al.* for the Cholesterol and Recurrent Events Trial Investigators (1996) Effect of pravastatin on coronary events after myocardial infarction in patients with average cholesterol levels. *NEJM.* **335**: 1001–9.

47 The Heart Outcomes Prevention Evaluation (HOPE) Study Investigators (2000) Effects of an angiotensin-converting enzyme inhibitor, ramipril, on cardiovascular events in high-risk patients. *NEJM.* **342**: 1445–53.

48 Heart Outcomes Prevention Evaluation (HOPE) Study Investigators (2000) Effects of ramipril on cardiovascular and microvascular outcomes in people with diabetes mellitus: results of the HOPE and MICRO-HOPE substudy. *Lancet.* **355**: 253–9.

49 Wood D, Durrington P, Poulter N *et al.* (1998) Joint British recommendations on prevention of coronary heart disease in clinical practice. *Heart.* **80 (supplement 2)**: S1–29.

50 Aspire Steering Group (1996) A British Cardiac Society survey of the potential for the secondary prevention of coronary heart disease: ASPIRE (action on secondary prevention through intervention to reduce events). *Heart.* **75**: 334–42.

51 Campbell NC, Thain J, George Deans H *et al.* (1998) Secondary prevention in coronary heart disease: baseline survey of provision in general practice. *BMJ.* **316**: 1430–44.

52 Campbell T (1998) The role of secondary prevention clinics. *BMJ.* **316**: 1434–7.

53 Robson J, Boomla K, Heart B *et al.* (2000) Estimating cardiovascular risk for primary prevention: outstanding questions for primary care. *BMJ.* **320**: 702–4.

54 Foord-Kelcey G (ed.) (2001) *Guidelines.* Medendium Group Publishing Ltd, Berkhamsted.

55 Office for National Statistics (2000) *Key Health Statistics from General Practice 1998.* Office for National Statistics, London.

56 Turner RC, Mills H, Neil HA *et al.* (1998) Risk factors for coronary heart disease in non-insulin-dependent diabetes mellitus: United Kingdom Prospective Diabetes Study. *BMJ.* **316**: 823–8.

57 Haq IU, Ramsey LE, Yeo WW *et al.* (1999) Is the Framingham risk function valid for Northern Europe populations? A comparison of methods estimating acute coronary risk in high-risk men. *Heart.* **81**: 40–6.

58 Downs JR, Cleofield M, Weis I *et al.* (1998) Primary prevention of acute coronary events with lovastatin in men and women with average cholesterol levels: results of AFCAPS/TexCAPS. Airforce Texas Coronary Atherosclerosis Prevention Study. *JAMA.* **279**: 1615–22.

59 Ramsay LE, Williams B, Johnston GD *et al.* (1999) Guidelines for management of hypertension: report of the third working party of the British Hypertension Society. *J Hum Hyperten.* **13**: 575.

60 Standing Medical Advisory Committee (1997) *The Use of Statins.* Department of Health, Leeds.

61 Campbell NC (1999) Edinburgh consensus conference on lipid lowering. *Trends Cardiol Vascular Dis.* **1**: 31–4.

62 West of Scotland Coronary Prevention Study Group (1998) Influence of pravastatin and plasma lipids on clinical events in the West of Scotland Coronary Prevention Study (WOSCOPS). *Circulation.* **97**: 1440–5.

63 Norris RM (2000) The GP's role in acute myocardial infarction. *Practitioner.* **244**: 510–37.

64 Pittard J (2000) *Pocket Guide. Post-MI care 2000.* Medical Imprint, London.

65 Collier J (ed.) (2000) Tackling myocardial infarction. *Drug Ther Bull.* **38**: 17–22.

66 de Bono D for the Joint Working Party of British Cardiac Society and Royal College of Physicians of London (1999) Investigation and management of stable angina: revised guidelines 1998. *Heart.* **81**: 546–55.

67 Scottish Intercollegiate Guidelines Network (1999) *Diagnosis and Treatment of Heart Failure Due to Left Ventricular Systolic Dysfunction.* Scottish Intercollegiate Guidelines Network Secretariat, Edinburgh.

68 McDonagh TA, Morrison CE, Lawrence A *et al.* (1997) Symptomatic and asymptomatic left ventricular systolic dysfunction in an urban population. *Lancet.* **350**: 829–33.

69 Hobbs FDR, Davis RC, McLeod S *et al.* (1998) Prevalence of heart failure in high-risk groups. *J Am Coll Cardiol.* **31 (Supplement 5)**: 85C (abstract).

70 Hobbs FDR (2000) Management of heart failure: evidence versus practice. Does current prescribing provide optimal treatment for heart failure? (Review article) *Br J Gen Pract.* **50**: 735–42.

71 Bonneux L, Barendregt J, Meeter K *et al.* (1994) Estimating clinical morbidity due to ischaemic heart disease and congestive heart failure: the future risk of heart failure. *Am J Public Health.* **84**: 20–8.

72 Eccles M, Freemantle N, Mason JM and the North of England ACE-Inhibitor Guideline Development Group, North of England Evidence-based Guideline Development Project (1998) Guideline for angiotensin-converting-enzyme inhibitors in primary care management of adults with symptomatic heart failure. *BMJ.* **316**: 1369–75.

73 Collier J (ed.) (2000) Heart failure drugs: what's new? *Drug Ther Bull.* **38**: 25–7.

74 Khunti K, Baker R and Grimshaw G (2000) Diagnosis of patients with chronic heart failure in primary care: usefulness of history, examination and investigations. *Br J Gen Pract.* **50**: 50–4.

75 Cleland JGF, McGowan J and Clark A (1999) The evidence for beta-blockers in heart failure equals or surpasses that for angiotensin-converting-enzyme inhibitors. *BMJ.* **318**: 824–5.

76 Strongburg A (1998) Heart failure clinics. *Heart.* **80**: 426–7.

77 Dunning M, Abi-Aad G, Gilbert D *et al.* (1999) *Experience, Evidence and Everyday Practice.* King's Fund, London.

78 Nielson OW, Hausen JF, Hilden J *et al.* (2000) Risk assessment of left ventricular systolic dysfunction in primary care: cross-sectional study evaluating a range of diagnostic tests. *BMJ.* **320**: 220–4.

79 Edinburgh Health Care Trust (1996) *Heart Manual.* Albert Gate Ltd, Grimsby.

80 British Heart Foundation (2000) *Cardiac Rehabilitation.* British Heart Foundation, London.

81 Hylek EM, Skates SJ, Sheehan MA *et al.* (1996) An analysis of the lowest effective intensity of prophylactic anticoagulation for patients with non-rheumatic atrial fibrillation. *NEJM.* **335**: 540–6.

82 Cobbe SM (1999) Atrial fibrillation in hospital and general practice: the Sir James McKenzie Centenary Consensus Conference. In: *Proceedings of the Royal College of Physicians of Edinburgh.* **29 (Supplement 6)**.

83 Campbell NC (1999) The role of secondary prevention clinics for CHD. *Trends Cardiol Vascular Dis.* **1**: 27–31.

84 Evens B and Primatesta P (eds) (1999) *Health Survey for England: cardiovascular disease '98.* Volume 1. Findings. The Stationery Office, London.

85 Cradduck G (1994) *Stroke and CHD Prevention by Therapeutic Intervention. Initiative 3 – the use of antithrombotic therapy in atrial fibrillation.* Northamptonshire Medical Audit Advisory Group, Northampton.

86 Office for National Statistics (1998) *Key Health Statistics from General Practice 1996.* Office for National Statistics, London.

Read codes for monitoring template for NSF for coronary heart disease

(Read codes will be replaced by SNOMED eventually – this System-atized Nomenclature of Medicine should be available in late 2001.)

Developed by East Staffordshire PCG and Queens Hospital Burton

Diagnosis

G3 . . .	IHD
G30 . .	Acute MI
G33 . .	Angina

Coronary artery procedures

7928 .	PTCA
792 . .	CABG

Cardiac conditions

G5730	Atrial fibrillation
G58 . .	Heart failure
G6 . . .	Cerebrovascular disease
G65 . .	Transient cerebral ischaemia
G73 . .	Peripheral vascular disease: artery/arteriole and capillary disease

Investigations

3213 .	Exercise stress test
32130	Normal
32131	Abnormal

321 . .	Resting ECG
	Normal Y/N
	Abnormal Y/N

Echocardiogram

| 58530 | Normal |
| 58531 | Abnormal |

Risk factors

137 . .	Smoking status
1371 .	Never smoked
137S .	Ex-smoker
137R .	Current smoker
6791 .	Advice given

C10 . .	Diabetes mellitus
C108 .	Insulin-dependent
C109 .	Non-insulin-dependent

14A2 .	Hypertension
2469 .	BP systolic
246A .	BP diastolic
44P . .	Serum cholesterol
44P1 .	Normal
44P2 .	Raised

22K . .	BMI
22K4	BMI 25–29 overweight
22K5	BMI 30+ obese

138 . .	Exercise
1385 .	Very active
1384 .	Moderate
1383 .	Light
1382 .	Inactive

136 . .	Alcohol
1361 .	Teetotaller
1364 .	Moderate drinker, 3–6 units per day
1365 .	Heavy drinker, 7–9 units per day
1366 .	Very heavy drinker, >9 units per day

Family history

Diagnosed CHD
12C2 .	Immediate family
Mother/sister	<65 years Y/N
Father/brother	<60 years Y/N

Hypertension
12C1 .	Immediate family
Mother/sister	<65 years Y/N
Father/brother	<60 years Y/N

CVA/stroke/TIA
12C4 .	Immediate family
Mother/sister	<65 years Y/N
Father/brother	<60 years Y/N

Symptom/angina control

662K0	Stable	
662K1	Poor	
662K2	Improving	} Picking list within template
662K3	Deteriorating	
662Kz	NOS	

Secondary prevention therapy

Health education
6791 .	Advice on smoking
6792 .	Advice on alcohol consumption
6798 .	Advice on exercise
6799 .	Advice on diet

8B28 .	Lipid-lowering therapy

8B63 .	Aspirin – includes over the counter
8124 .	Aspirin contraindication

8B69 .	Beta-blocker prophylaxis
8162 .	Beta-blocker not indicated
8B6B .	ACE-inhibitor prophylaxis

ZV579	Cardiac rehabilitation

662N .	Recall

Prevalence data for a range of conditions relating to coronary heart disease

Table A2.1 Expected number of cardiovascular conditions for a sample practice of 10 000 patients with an age–sex distribution that mirrors the population of England

		Number of patients		
		Men	Women	Total
Expected number of patients who are smoking – current		1150	1140	2290
Expected number of patients with hypertension[84]	Pre-1998 definition*	630	750	1380
	Post-1998 definition*	1480	1320	2800
Expected number of patients with diabetes		70	60	130
Expected number of patients with atrial fibrillation (MAAG Northamptonshire)[85]		50	60	110
Expected number of patients who have ever had a heart attack		140	70	210
Expected number of patients who have ever had angina		190	160	350
Expected number of patients with IHD (MI and angina)		250	190	440
Expected number of patients who have ever had a stroke		80	70	150
Expected number of patients with IHD or stroke (MI, angina or stroke)		290	270	560
Expected number of patients with heart failure	Lower limit	50	50	100
	Upper limit	100	100	200
Expected 30% risk of cardiac event over 10 years[53]		70	70	140

Source: Health Survey for England, 1999.[84]
* Includes treated and untreated hypertension.
Pre-1998 informants were considered to be hypertensive if their systolic blood pressure was 160 mmHg or over, or their diastolic blood pressure was 95 mmHg or over, or they were taking medication that affects blood pressure.
After 1998 informants were considered to be hypertensive if their systolic blood pressure was 140 mmHg or over, or their diastolic blood pressure was 90 mmHg or over, or they were taking medication that affects blood pressure.

Table A2.2 Expected number of patients who are current smokers for a sample practice of 10 000 patients with an age–sex distribution that mirrors the population of England

Age (years)	Number of current smokers		
	Men	Women	Total
< 15	0	0	0
15–24	250	40	290
25–34	290	100	390
35–44	230	170	400
45–54	180	230	410
55–64	110	230	340
65–74	70	210	280
≥ 75	20	160	180
Total	1150	1140	2290

Source: Health Survey for England, 1999.[84]

Table A2.3 Expected number of patients with hypertension (pre-1998 definition – *see* page 153) for a sample practice of 10 000 patients with an age–sex distribution that mirrors the population of England

Age (years)	Number of patients		
	Men	Women	Total
< 15	0	0	0
15–24	10	0	10
25–34	10	10	20
35–44	60	30	90
45–54	110	90	200
55–64	160	140	300
65–74	160	220	380
≥ 75	120	260	380
Total	630	750	1380

Source: Health Survey for England, 1999.[84]

Table A2.4 Expected number of patients with hypertension (post-1998 definition – *see* page 153) for a sample practice of 10 000 patients with an age-sex distribution that mirrors the population of England

	Number of patients		
Age (years)	*Men*	*Women*	*Total*
< 15	0	0	0
15–24	100	20	120
25–34	160	50	210
35–44	190	90	280
45–54	280	200	480
55–64	290	260	550
65–74	270	330	600
≥ 75	190	370	560
Total	1480	1320	2800

Source: Health Survey for England, 1999.[84]

Table A2.5 Expected number of patients with diabetes for a sample practice of 10 000 patients with an age–sex distribution that mirrors the population of England

	Number of patients		
Age (years)	*Men*	*Women*	*Total*
< 15	0	0	0
15–24	0	0	0
25–34	0	0	0
35–44	10	10	20
45–54	10	10	20
55–64	20	10	30
65–74	20	20	40
75–84	10	10	20
≥ 85	0	0	0
Total	70	60	130

Source: Office for National Statistics, 1998.[86]

Table A2.6 Expected number of patients with atrial fibrillation for a sample practice of 10 000 patients with an age–sex distribution that mirrors the population of England

Age (years)	Number of patients		
	Men	Women	Total
< 65	10	10	20
65–74	10	10	20
≥ 75	30	40	70
Total	50	60	110

Source: G Cradduck, Northamptonshire Medical Audit Advisory Group, 1994.[85]

Table A2.7 Expected number of patients who have ever had a heart attack for a sample practice of 10 000 patients with an age–sex distribution that mirrors the population of England

Age (years)	Number of patients		
	Men	Women	Total
< 15	0	0	0
15–24	0	0	0
25–34	0	0	0
35–44	0	0	0
45–54	20	10	30
55–64	40	10	50
65–74	40	20	60
≥ 75	40	30	70
Total	140	70	210

Source: Health Survey for England, 1999.[84]

Table A2.8 Expected number of patients who have ever had angina for a sample practice of 10 000 patients with an age–sex distribution that mirrors the population of England

| Age (years) | Number of patients | | |
	Men	Women	Total
< 15	0	0	0
15–24	0	0	0
25–34	0	0	0
35–44	10	0	10
45–54	20	10	30
55–64	50	30	80
65–74	60	40	100
≥ 75	50	80	130
Total	190	160	350

Source: Health Survey for England, 1999.[84]

Table A2.9 Expected number of patients with IHD* for a sample practice of 10 000 patients with an age–sex distribution mirroring the population of England

| Age (years) | Number of patients | | |
	Men	Women	Total
< 15	0	0	0
15–24	0	0	0
25–34	0	0	0
35–44	10	0	10
45–54	30	10	40
55–64	70	30	100
65–74	80	60	140
≥ 75	60	90	150
Total	250	190	440

Source: Health Survey for England, 1999.[84]
* Ischaemic heart disease, reported as doctor-diagnosed heart attack or angina.

Table A2.10 Expected number of patients who have ever had a stroke for a sample practice of 10 000 patients with an age–sex distribution that mirrors the population of England

| Age (years) | Number of patients | | |
	Men	Women	Total
< 15	0	0	0
15–24	0	0	0
25–34	0	0	0
35–44	0	0	0
45–54	10	0	10
55–64	20	10	30
65–74	20	20	40
≥ 75	30	40	70
Total	80	70	150

Source: Health Survey for England, 1999.[84]

Table A2.11 Expected number of patients with IHD* or stroke for a sample practice of 10 000 patients with an age–sex distribution that mirrors the population of England

| Age (years) | Number of patients | | |
	Men	Women	Total
< 15	0	0	0
15–24	0	0	0
25–34	0	10	10
35–44	10	10	20
45–54	30	20	50
55–64	80	40	120
65–74	90	70	160
≥ 75	80	120	200
Total	290	270	560

Source: Health Survey for England, 1999.[84]
* Ischaemic heart disease, reported as doctor-diagnosed heart attack or angina.

Table A2.12 Number of individuals expected to have a 30% or higher risk of a cardiac event over 10 years for a sample practice of 10 000 patients with an age–sex distribution that mirrors the population of England

Age (years)	Number of patients		
	Men	Women	Total
< 35	0	0	0
35–69	70	70	140
70–75	0	0	0
Total	70	70	140

Source: J Robson *et al.*, 2000.[53]

National Service Framework for Coronary Heart Disease – extracts

Standards

Standards 1 and 2: reducing heart disease in the population

1 *The NHS and partner agencies should* develop, implement and monitor policies that reduce the prevalence of coronary risk factors in the population, and reduce inequalities in risks of developing heart disease.
2 *The NHS and partner agencies should* contribute to a reduction in the prevalence of smoking in the local population.

Standards 3 and 4: preventing CHD in high-risk patients

3 *General practitioners and primary healthcare teams should* identify all people with established cardiovascular disease and offer them comprehensive advice and appropriate treatment to reduce their risks.
4 *General practitioners and primary healthcare teams should* identify all people at significant risk of cardiovascular disease but who have not developed symptoms, and offer them appropriate advice and treatment to reduce their risks.

Standards 5, 6 and 7: heart attack and other acute coronary syndromes

5 *People with symptoms of a possible heart attack should* receive help from an individual equipped with and appropriately trained in the use of a defibrillator within 8 minutes of calling for help, to maximise the benefits of resuscitation should it be necessary.

6 *People thought to be suffering from a heart attack should* be assessed professionally and, if indicated, receive aspirin. Thrombolysis should be given within 60 minutes of calling for professional help.

7 *NHS trusts should* put in place agreed protocols/systems of care so that people admitted to hospital with proven heart attack are appropriately assessed and offered treatments of proven clinical and cost-effectiveness to reduce their risk of disability and death.

Standard 8: stable angina

8 *People with symptoms of angina or suspected angina should* receive appropriate investigation and treatment to relieve their pain and reduce their risk of coronary events.

Standards 9 and 10: revascularisation

9 *People with angina that is increasing in frequency or severity should* be referred to a cardiologist urgently or, for those at greatest risk, as an emergency.

10 *NHS trusts should* put in place hospital-wide systems of care so that patients with suspected or confirmed coronary heart disease receive timely and appropriate investigation and treatment to relieve their symptoms and reduce their risk of subsequent coronary events.

Standard 11: heart failure

11 *Doctors should* arrange for people with suspected heart failure to be offered appropriate investigations (e.g. electrocardiography, echocardiography) that will confirm or refute the diagnosis. For those in whom heart failure is confirmed, its cause should be

identified, and treatments that are most likely both to relieve their symptoms and to reduce their risk of death should be offered.

Standard 12: cardiac rehabilitation

12 *NHS trusts should* put in place agreed protocols/systems of care so that, prior to leaving hospital, people admitted to hospital suffering from coronary heart disease have been invited to participate in a multidisciplinary programme of secondary prevention and cardiac rehabilitation. The aim of the programme will be to reduce their risk of subsequent cardiac problems, and to promote their return to a full and normal life.

Timetable for all organisations: organisational and health promotion milestones and goals

Date	Health promotion and general organisation
October 2000	HAs, LAs, PCGs/PCTs and NHS trusts will: • have actively participated in the development of health improvement programmes (HImPs) • have agreed their responsibilities for and contributions to specific projects identified in HImPs • have agreed a mechanism for being held to account for the actions that they have agreed to deliver as part of the HImP • have agreed a mechanism for ensuring that progress on health promotion policies is reported to and reviewed by the Board • have identified a link person to be a point of contact for partner agencies
April 2001	HAs, LAs, PCGs/PCTs and NHS trusts will: • have agreed and be contributing to the delivery of the local programme of effective policies on (a) reducing smoking, (b) promoting healthy eating, (c) increasing physical activity and (d) reducing overweight and obesity • have a mechanism for ensuring that all new policies and all existing policies which are subject to review can be screened for health impacts

Date	Health promotion and general organisation
April 2001 (cont.)	• as an employer, have implemented a policy on smoking • be able to refer clients/service users to specialist smoking cessation services, including clinics • have produced an equity profile and set local equity targets
April 2002	*HAs, LAs, PCGs/PCTs and NHS trusts will:* • have quantitative data no more than 12 months old about the implementation of the policies on: – reducing the prevalence of smoking – promoting healthy eating – promoting physical activity – reducing overweight and obesity • as an employer, have developed 'green' transport plans and taken steps to implement employee-friendly policies
April 2003	*HAs, LAs, PCGs/PCTs and NHS trusts will:* • have implemented plans to evaluate progress against national targets associated with *Saving Lives: Our Healthier Nation* and local targets.
NSF goal	• contribute to the target reduction in deaths from circulatory diseases as outlined in *Saving Lives: Our Healthier Nation* of up to 200 000 lives in total by 2010

Timetable for primary care: milestones and goals

Date	Primary care	Stable angina	Heart failure
October 2000	Clinical teams should meet as a team at least once every quarter to plan and discuss the results of clinical audit, and to discuss clinical issues generally. PCGs/PCTs and hospitals that together form a local network of cardiac care should have effective means for agreeing an integrated system for quality assessment and quality improvement		
April 2001	All medical records and hospital correspondence must be held in a way that allows them to be retrieved readily in order of date. Appropriate medical records must contain easily discernible drug-therapy lists for patients on long-term therapy		

Date	Primary care	Stable angina	Heart failure
April 2001 (cont.)	A systematically developed and maintained practice-based CHD register is in place and actively used to provide structured care to people with CHD		A systematically developed and maintained practice-based CHD register is in place and actively used to provide structured care to people with CHD
April 2002	A protocol describing the systematic assessment, treatment and follow-up of patients with CHD has been agreed locally and is used to provide structured care to patients with CHD		A protocol describing the systematic assessment, treatment and follow-up of patients with heart failure has been agreed locally and is used to provide structured care to patients with heart failure
April 2003	Clinical audit data no more than 12 months old are available that describe the use of relevant effective interventions in primary care	Clinical audit data no more than 12 months old are available that describe the use of relevant effective interventions in angina	Clinical audit data no more than 12 months old are available that describe the use of relevant effective interventions in heart failure
NSF goals	Every practice should offer advice about each of the specified interventions to those in whom they are indicated, demonstrated by clinical audit data no more than 12 months old	Every practice should offer advice about each of the specified interventions to those in whom they are indicated, demonstrated by clinical audit data no more than 12 months old	Every primary care team should ensure that all those with heart failure are receiving a full package of appropriate investigation and treatment, demonstrated by clinical audit data no more than 12 months old

Sources of information and support: organisations, websites, self-help groups and training programmes

Evidence-based resources

Agency for Health Care Policy and Research (AHCPR):
  http://www.ahcpr.gov

Bandolier: http://ebandolier.com
  The Bandolier site summarises the issues surrounding smoking cessation
  in a simple text format.

Canadian Medical Association: http://www.cma.ca/cpgs/

Cochrane Collaboration: http://www.cochrane.org
  The Cochrane review offers an index of general resources on smoking.

eGuidelines: http://www.eguidelines.co.uk

Guideline Appraisal Project: http://www.cche.net/principles/content_all.asp

Guideline Project: http://www.ihs.ox.ac.uk/guidelines/

HoN (Health on the Net): http://www.hon.ch

Medline: http://www.omni.ac.uk/medline

New Zealand Guidelines Group: http://www.nzgg.org.nz/

NLM Health Services: http://www.nlm.nih.gov

North of England Evidence-Based Guidelines: http://www.ncl.ac.uk/
  ~ncenthsr/publicn/publicn.htm

OMNI (Organising Medical Networked Information):
http://www.omni.ac.uk

Pathways to the NSF: http://www.nsfpathways.co.uk/
nsf_pathways_homepage.html

PRODIGY: http://www.prodigy.nhs.uk

Scottish Intercollegiate Guidelines Network (SIGN):
http://www.sign.ac.uk

St George's Health Care Evaluation Unit:
http://www.sghms.ac.uk/depts/phs/hceu/nhsguide.htm

UK Health Centre: http://www.healthcentre.org.uk/hc/library/
guidelines.htm

WISDOM Centre: http://www.wisdomnet.co.uk

Official documents

http://www.official-documents.co.uk/document/doh/tobacco/contents.htm
A quick route to the many official documents, including a list of hyperlinks
papers behind the national strategy.

US sites

http://www.stop-smoking-secrets.com/
http://www.surgeongeneral.gov/tobacco/
http://www.cdc.gov/tobacco/

Relevant organisations

Action Heart
Wellesley House, 117 Wellington Road, Dudley DY1 1UB.
Tel: 01384 230222.

British Heart Foundation
14 Fitzharding Street, London W1H 4DH.
Tel: 020 7935 0185. Fax: 020 7486 1273. Website: www.bhf.org.uk

British Hyperlipidaemia Association
c/o David Middleton Communications, Environmental Business Centre,
B & IC, Aston Science Park, Birmingham B7 4BJ.
Tel: 0121 693 8338. Fax: 0121 693 8448. Email: ebc@dircon.co.uk

British Hypertension Society
Information Service, 127 High Street, Teddington, Middlesex TW11 8HH.
Tel: 020 8977 0012. Fax: 020 8977 0055.

Diabetes UK
7th Floor, Elizabeth House, 22 Suffolk Street, Queensway, Birmingham
B1 1LS.
Tel: 0121 643 5488. Fax: 0121 633 4399. Email: bda@dial.pipex.com

Family Heart Association
PO Box 303, Maidenhead, Berks SL6 9UX.
Tel: 01628 628638.

Health Education Board of Scotland (HEBS)
http://www.hebs.scot.nhs.uk
The Scottish equivalent of the Health Development Agency site has many
graphics and animations.

Scottish Heart and Arterial Risk Prevention (SHARP) Group
Department of Medicine, Ninewells Hospital and Medical School, Dundee
DD1 9SY.
Tel: 01382 660111. Fax: 01382 660675.
Email: srmcewan@ninewells.dundee.ac.uk

Tobacco Campaign Helpline Service
Tel: 0800 1690169.

Coronary heart disease websites

UK

ASH (Action on Smoking and Health)
http://www.ash.org.uk

BBC Education Heart Special
http://www.bbc.co.uk/health/

Blood Pressure Association
http://www.bpassoc.org.uk

British Cardiac Patients Association
http://www.cardiac-bcpa.co.uk/index.html

British Cardiac Society
http://www.bcs.com/

British Heart Foundation (BHF)
http://www.bhf.org.uk/

British Heart Foundation Statistics Database
http://www.dphpc.ox.ac.uk/bhfhprg/stats/index.html

British Hypertension Society
http://www.hyp.ac.uk/bhs/

Cardiac Rehabilitation
http://www.cardiacrehabilitation.org.uk/

Cardiomyopathy Association
http://www.cardiomyopathy.org/homepage.htm

Chest, Heart and Stroke, Scotland
http://www.chss.org.uk/

Children's Heart Federation
http://www.childrens-heart-fed.org.uk/

Coronary Prevention Group
http://www.healthnet.org.uk/new/cpg/index.htm

Giving Up Smoking
http://www.givingupsmoking.co.uk/
This is another national site, backed by the NHS, designed for those trying to give up smoking rather than for professionals.

GUCH – Grown-Up Congenital Heart Patients Association
http://www.guch.demon.co.uk/index.htm

Heart (Journal)
http://heart.bmjjournals.com/

Heart Link Support Group
http://www.heartlink.org.uk/

National Heart Forum
http://www.heartforum.org.uk/nationalheartforum.html

Quit Smoking UK
http://www.quitsmokinguk.com
This is a more professional site – an entire portal devoted entirely to those trying to quit.

Resuscitation Council UK
http://www.resus.org.uk/SiteIndx.htm

Europe

European Heart Journal
http://www.harcourt-international.com/journals/euhj/

European Heart Network
http://www.ehnheart.org/

European Society of Cardiology
http://www.escardio.org/

USA

Adult Congenital Heart Association
http://www.achaheart.org/

American Heart Association
http://www.americanheart.org/

American Hypertension Society
http://www.ash-us.org/

Circulation (Journal)
http://circ.ahajournals.org/

Heart Information Network
http://www.heartinfo.org/

HeartPoint
http://www.heartpoint.com/

National Heart, Lung and Blood Institute
http://www.nhlbi.nih.gov/index.htm

The Heart: An Online Exploration
http://sln.fi.edu/biosci/heart.html

World-wide

Coronary Health Care (Journal)
http://www.harcourt-international.com/journals/chec/default.cfm

Global Cardiology Network
http://www.globalcardiology.org/

International Society for Heart Research
http://www.ishrworld.org/

World Heart Day
http://www.worldheartday.com/

World Heart Federation
http://www.worldheart.org/

World Hypertension League
http://www.mco.edu/whl/

Training programmes

The **British Heart Foundation** runs a programme of training in the secondary prevention of coronary heart disease for nurses working in the community. It is accredited by Buckinghamshire Chilterns University College for 30 CATS points at Level 2.

Apply to the BHF Heart Save Project, University of Oxford, Institute of Health Sciences, Old Road, Headington, Oxford OX3 7LF. Tel: 01865 226975. Fax: 01865 226739. Email: heartsave@dphpc.ox.ac.uk

The **Scottish Heart and Arterial Risk Prevention (SHARP)** course for nurses includes cardiovascular risk: identification, stratification and management.

Contact the SHARP Office, University Department of Medicine, Ninewells Hospital and Medical School, Dundee DD1 9SY. Tel: 01382 660111 ext 33124.

The **British Hypertension Society** Information Service gives advice about local courses in hypertension and CHD risk factors.

Tel: 020 8725 3412. Fax: 020 8725 2959.

Index